For more information
NaturoMedic™.com   Phone: (905) 684-4934
296 Welland Avenue   Fax: (905) 684-1849
St. Catharines, Ontario   Email: info@naturomedic.com
L2R 7L9   Website: www.NaturoMedic.com

1

To our patients for working alongside us in our pursuit of knowledge. Your devotion and patience has been invaluable. Thank you for the challenge and giving us the opportunity to rise to the occasion.

To our families for their endless support, love and guidance. Thank you to our prayer warriors for their diligence and unwavering persistence.

"Keep your dreams alive. Understand to achieve anything requires faith and belief in yourself, vision, hard work, determination, and dedication. Remember all things are possible for those who believe."
–Gail Devers

Contributors

Dr. Erin MacKimmie ND, RN BNSc.

Joanna Barnett B.A.

Acknowledgments

We would like to thank Diana Taylor, Rayan Mokbel BHSc, MaryAnn Magnotta RN BA CNCC (C), and Silvia Magnotta BA RMT SIT for their support, patience and persistence in providing us with insightful feedback to manifest this book.

A message from Dr. Michael A. Prytula ND.

...The medical doctors were perplexed. The large muscles throughout this former high school athlete's body were deteriorating and losing function. His weight had plummeted from 165 lbs. to 100 lbs. in less than 2 months. Acne and infection had ravaged his skin, changing its colour and contours on a daily basis. His large muscle groups were paralyzed while his small muscle groups, like his hands, were still functional. He could still get up and go to the washroom, but it was an arduously painful 20-30 minutes to make the 40 step roundtrip. The medical doctors from the University Hospital had performed an experiment by giving this young man a huge dose of corticosteroids for his cystic acne condition. Did this experiment go awfully wrong? Did this young man have Parkinson's Disease? Multiple Sclerosis? Polio? Muscular Dystrophy? A Spinal cord tumour? Brain tumour? ALS? Guillian-Barre syndrome? Or Flesh eating disease? The list of possibilities was exhausting. But one thing was certain; he was deteriorating. His mother, by his bedside, faithfully prayed for a miracle as his precipitous decline continued...

That was 1980. Not the way my family and I desired to spend Christmas. I questioned if this was the intended purpose for my life. This self-centered proud young man was intending to be in the military with aspirations of becoming a helicopter pilot. I certainly did not think my future was medicine but, in hindsight, God had other plans. With hope seemingly lost, out of desperation, I prayed to my mother's God asking Him to do with me what He wanted. I could not live like this, in this corpse of a body. This was not living; this was barely existing. As I wallowed in defeat, wishing I was not there, my prayer warrior mother was receiving her miracle and mine. I was becoming better. Much to my surprise and that of the doctors and staff I was getting stronger, moving faster, talking faster and becoming engaged again. Soon I was discharged from the hospital with the arduous task of recovery. Much to my amazement, recovery was swift. But healing was not complete by any means! Fatigue was the norm. Muscle control and strength were wanting. Something was still wrong, significantly wrong. The quest for healing and health continued. Internal medicine specialists, neurologists, and infectious disease specialist—no one had answers. Or else the explanation was ludicrous, basically saying "it's all in your head".

This path of discovery exposed the gaps in mainstream medicine. I was no longer sick enough to qualify. I pursued the path less travelled. Nutrition therapy, botanical medicine, chiropractic adjustments, acupuncture and other therapies were added to the list of what did not work for me. Some therapies were not next door, so driving 8 hours one way to have a doctor's visit was not out of the norm. Finally, as the exhausted list of treatments grew, homeopathy presented itself. Dr.

Ed, a homeopath in his 80s with a twinkle in his eyes, gave me hope, knowledge and wisdom. "Take this and you are going to feel worse for the first few days and then better", a phrase I have since shared during over 100,000 patient visits. His prognosis was accurate. I felt awful, with an unending migraine and extreme fatigue that was relentless over four days. On the fifth day I received my second miracle breakthrough. All my symptoms were improving and not just in small amounts. I was high as a kite. I felt amazing. My enthusiasm for this new medicine was infectious and my new found health was on display for all to see. I was back.

It was then that it was decided that this was the path for me. Dr. Ed's encouragement and direction pointed me to Naturopathic Medicine—an old but new field of healing. A minimum of seven years of schooling was a rather overwhelming idea to an underachieving academic, but passion overcame. However the path of healing and obtaining optimum health can be a fickle one. I started to deteriorate again, thankfully not as severely as before. At this point, I was about to try something different. Very different and out of the norm for an initiated member of the consumer generation—a fast. I was committed. Seven days and no food while taking supplements to ensure proper detox. Detox I did. Headaches, body aches, vomiting, diarrhea! Then on day four, miracle number three exposed itself. I was back and high as a kite again! But this time I needed answers. How come I felt so awful and then better? What was going on? I asked the easily available MD's what was going on and they could not offer an explanation. Dr. Ed's wisdom once again revealed a health mystery, the concept of the healing crisis.

The quest for health, in this case optimum health, continued through three years of premed university and four years at Naturopathic College. Upon graduation, this idealistic, newly crowned Naturopath was released into the world. Naively thinking that all things could be cured with the tools I was trained in, I quickly reached the limitations of my training and needed more tools. To accelerate my learning curve and to keep costs down for patients, I chose to develop a high volume practice. This way I could also see what technique or therapy was working and what was not working very quickly. I rapidly expanded my practice into IV therapeutics as some patients' digestive tracts could not absorb nutrients for healing. I had heard about different treatments for heart disease and AIDS as well. IV chelation for vascular disease and IV Ozone for infections and immune suppressed diseases were added to my practices' pharmacopeia. In pursuit of these treatments, my quest for optimum health was derailed as the political nature of these therapies was exposed and the following legal battles took their tolls. My former prolonged use of cortisone during the treatment of my paralysis in combination with the stress precipitated a diagnosis of ulcerative colitis. At the

5

same time, I had a number of patients present with an inability to digest foods, food allergies and surprisingly allergies to nutrients. Just to round things out, a number of menopausal ladies presented with osteoporosis. Surprisingly, they could not take calcium supplements. In fact they reacted severely to calcium supplements with migraines, fatigue, diarrhea and vomiting. These reactions caused me to rethink my health strategy at the time. What was going on? Even more importantly, how could I fix it? This is when NAET, the precursor to the EAT, was introduced.

EATs, stress management and IV nutrients all helped hold my condition in check and healed a lot of my patients. After seeing some of the limits of these therapies, patients again presented with a disease causing factor for which I needed to find an effective tool to address it. Subconscious emotions were the common theme with these patients and this resulted in a number of cures, but the treatment process was arduous. I needed to shorten it so that I still had time to address other factors in a doctor's visit. Hence Mental Reprogramming Technique came into being. This retained all the benefits of the various subconscious techniques and put them into a process that was amazingly efficient and effective. This technique helped patients immensely and some incredible miracles were witnessed by staff and I. Next, microorganisms and infection seemed to be the common issue but not just any type of infection—stealth infections. This sequence of events then presented itself over and over again as various disease causing factors were uncovered and treatments to address them effectively.

As I have gone through this process of discovery with our patients and with my own health, I have been blessed to witness many miracles and cures. When Dr. Mike Um arrived to join my practice in 2002, my determination was starting to crumble. Through his support, we persisted and ultimately developed many tools for doctors to use and techniques to address factors where there was no previous treatment. All these processes have culminated in identifying the many disease causing factors that are being addressed in this book. Dr. Mary Magnotta ND joined our team initially as a student in 2008. Dr. Erin MacKimmie ND joined NaturoMedic.com in 2010. They all have been an asset to the NaturoMedic.com team and their knowledge has contributed to our vision of health.

Our health strategy, The Health Continuum™, The Health Cup Analogy™ and The Weakest Link™ have all been developed to explain a strategy that works. We are thankful to our many patients for their determination to see results and for their willingness to let us utilize various treatments to isolate different factors and ensure results.

Table of Contents

Looking for a Miracle?

In many ways we are all looking and waiting for a miracle, whether it is a health miracle, financial miracle, relationship miracle, etc. Who would not love the freedom of winning the lottery? But what exactly is a miracle? According to the Merriam-Webster dictionary, a miracle is an extraordinary event manifesting divine intervention in human affairs.

In a miracle, the responsibility lies on another party. In other words, there is nothing required of us and the miracle is provided by something/someone else. As appreciative as many of us would be of a miracle, what truly is the extent of our benefit and how much have we really learned? Statistics have shown that lottery recipients of $50,000 to $150,000 are more likely to file for bankruptcy in the three to five years afterwards. Winners chose not to pay off any of their debt, failing to learn from their experience. Their behavior did not change, only the amount of money temporarily in their bank account.

Similar parallels may be drawn for recipients of healing miracles. Consider the man who, when given a second chance with an artificial/new heart, was met in the recovery room with a hot dog and a beer before being subsequently wheeled outside for a cigarette. It is difficult to question whether this person was particularly appreciative of their miracle. It is evident that they did not deviate from any behavior that led to their current circumstance. It is well-known that the survival rate of people who have successfully quit smoking following coronary bypass improves significantly compared to persistent smokers. Only 39% of smoker's grafts are disease free after 5 years as opposed to 52% of nonsmokers. Self-improvement is essential to the long-term benefits of your miracle. These statistics beg the question of **whether we need a miracle to change our lives or can we initiate changes independently of divine intervention?**

While many may continue to wait for their "miracle cure" or "miracle drug", you can begin shifting your understanding of health and the paradigm of a miracle. You can be blessed with good health! So what is the difference between a miracle cure and being blessed with good health? **A strategy, will power and a willingness to change are the three tools you need to begin making a difference in your future.** A miracle is usually a one shot deal; however, the blessings of good health are infinite.

The Chinese proverb "Give a man a fish and you feed him for a day. Teach a man to fish and you feed him for a lifetime" is a good example of being blessed with good health. By providing knowledge of a new skill, the man is now able to provide for himself and his family long-term and therefore is not always relying

12

on another party to do the work. Knowledge is empowerment. Understanding the responsibility you have for your life and your health will make a difference on your road to success. The Health Navigator provides education on the disease factors contributing to your health status and helps you discover which treatments are right for your path to success. The lessons of the Navigator are waiting for the one ready to make a dedication to themselves and to their health. Therefore instead of waiting to see which cards you are dealt next; let's start designing your own deck of cards.

Are you ready to be blessed with good health?

References:
1. http://www.merriam-webster.com/dictionary/miracle
2. Hoekstra, M. & Skiba, P.M. The Ticket to Easy Street? The Financial Consequences of Winning the Lottery Scott Hankins, University of Kentucky. Vanderbilt University Published on October 4, 2009
3. Voors AA, van Brussel BL, Plokker HW, et al. Smoking and cardiac events after venous coronary bypass surgery: a 15-year follow-up study. Circulation 1996; 93:42–7.
4. FitzGibbon GM, Leach AJ, Kafka HP. Atherosclerosis of coronary artery bypass grafts and smoking. CMAJ 1987;136:45
5. http://www.besancon-cardio.org/recommandations/cabg.pdf
6. International Thesaurus of Quotations, ed. Rhoda Thomas Tripp, p. 76, no. 3 (1970).

How to use this book

This book is organized into two sections. In Part I, each chapter focuses on specific disease causing factors associated with the Environment, Lifestyle, Body, Mind and Spirit. The first section is designed to identify the obstacles impeding your health.

Begin with Chapter 1 and 2 to start your journey and understand the unique strategy the Health Navigator offers. As you continue through the first section each chapter will introduce a variety of factors pertaining to one of the five main disease categories. There is a wealth of information available for the individual causes and some are very explicit with statistics. Although one can benefit from reading through each cause alone, we recommend that you focus on those that immediately relate to you. The understanding you develop in Part I will be built upon in later chapters along with therapeutic techniques.

As an additional bonus, NaturoMedic.com will be offering a free online accessible tool to help you build your own health profile. The site will provide a variety of questionnaires to assist you in determining which disease causing factors are important to you. Please refer to www.MyHealthNavigator.info. The website will continue to grow, with more options and knowledge as they become available.

The second section of the book is your road map to success. Part II outlines specific treatments to remove the disease causing factors and improve your well-being. The understanding attained from the multitude of therapies will undoubtedly provide answers to what is right for your path. We suggest that you begin reading those that correspond with your disease causing factors and you find to be most intriguing. These health-enhancing changes take time so try not to feel overwhelmed by the task. We know you can succeed. Thousands of patients have been blessed with good health from our unique strategy and treatments. Now we bring this program to you. It is your turn.

"What you do today can improve all your tomorrows."

--Ralph Marston

Part I: Identifying Obstacles

Chapter 1

Your Health Strategy

Your Health Strategy

Empowerment begins with you. The road through life is a winding path, filled with ups, downs, curves and twists. Multiple challenges and potholes will threaten your way. Having a road map to navigate the most direct route is essential.

The road through life is unmistakeably dependent upon your health. The strength and vigor of the mind, body and spirit are essential components that demand attention. Similar to regular oil changes and car maintenance, self-care is a priority that allows you to run optimally to face the obstacles ahead. Do not wait for your body to make a "noise" or start "leaking" before you take it in; take care of your health now. In the long-term, you cannot trade yourself in or buy a new one.

The Health Navigator is the road map designed to help you reach your health destination. It exposes the many potholes and obstacles you may encounter throughout your journey. The tools of the navigator will teach you to conquer the challenges of health on your road through life. Assessing your health status is the first step on your path to success.

What are your health goals?

Has anyone ever asked you what your **health goals** are? If they did, what would you say?

I would like:

- more energy
- improved sleep
- live pain free
- exercise more
- eat healthier
- better digestion

- live longer
- female wellness
- allergy free
- be disease free
- increased clarity of thought
- no pharmaceuticals

Goals are a powerful and critical tool in your health journey. They keep you on course, provide direction and facilitate focus. Setting goals provides each of us with a personal challenge and enforces health-conscience behaviours.

The human brain is not only designed to function in a goal oriented pattern it actually thirsts for the power of objectives. An estimated 10% of the brain's full capacity is consciously employed on a regular basis. The remaining 90% is subconscious, although goals have the ability to harness this latent potential. Chemicals, known as neurotransmitters, perform daily tasks within the brain. Dopamine is released when goals are set, acting as a motivator and rewarding us when we achieve the desired outcome. The neurotransmitter helps control pleasure centers in the brain, encouraging a repeat of rewarding behaviours (habits). Having a healthy goal (a successful habit) is a great objective to become addicted to.

The potential of the brain to aid in maintaining goals is a crucial asset. The billion bits of information the brain constantly receives every second is selectively filtered. The Reticular Activating System (RAS) is the area of the brain responsible for this process. It decides what to accept or reject. When goals are set the RAS becomes activated to notice opportunities that will help in achieving your endeavor.

Taking care of you is not a luxury—it is a necessity. Writing down concrete goals makes you responsible and accountable to develop successful habits. There is a detrimental cost to not taking action. You are not expendable and devotion to quality of life should be high on your priority list. Your physical, mental and spiritual state is begging for a commitment…it is time to set your starting point.

What are you currently doing & how is that working for you?

Are you happy with your health? Are you getting results? Evaluating your current situation is an essential part of setting goals. Ask yourself what it is you really want to achieve. **Disease treatment? Symptomatic relief? Disease prevention? Health optimization?**

The importance of the outcome is one of the key factors facilitating your commitment to your goals. A study by Gail Matthews from the Dominican University revealed some interesting conclusions about the benefits of setting goals. Matthews assigned volunteers from a broad range of ages and backgrounds to five different groups. Each group was asked to determine goals for a four-week time period; some were to just think about them; some were to write their goals down and others were asked to write progress reports to a friend as they completed their goals. The group that was asked to write down their goals had 50% more success in completing them than those who were only asked to think about their goals. The group that was asked to be accountable to a friend for completing their goals saw the highest level of success by fulfilling 76% of their stated goals. These conclusions suggest that writing out goals and being accountable to keep them are a great way to achieve the things we want to do. For goals to be effective, summary feedback that reveals progress is a key component to your strategy.

Time will always be critical in your long-term success. Staying on track, finding availability and remaining motivated with your busy schedule are constant challenges. Learning to prioritize is important. The brain will routinely filter out

18

goal-irrelevant activities so set specific goals to enhance your performance. Discovering the appropriate strategy is critical to achieving complex objectives.

"The greatest danger for most of us is not that our aim is too high and we miss it, but that it is too low and we reach it." - Michelangelo

What is your Health Strategy?

Has anyone ever asked you if you had a health strategy? Some of us have detailed strategies in place for how we plan to achieve success in our careers, security in our financial position or comfort in our retirement years. But how many of us have really thought about the need to create a personal **health strategy** that will allow us to enjoy all of these other achievements?

For most of us, our health strategy is a reactive one. We do not think about our health until something goes wrong. We can happily go for months or even years without seeing a health professional until an ache or pain warns us that something is not quite right. At that point, we schedule an appointment with our general practitioner (medical doctor). He/she does some blood work or possibly takes an x-ray or ultrasound of the problem area. After reviewing the results and doing other investigations, the practitioner makes a diagnosis and sends us on our way, possibly with some medication to treat the issue. We leave with the hope that it will be months or years before we need to see the doctor again.

But is this really a successful health strategy? Our bodies (and their proper functioning physically, mentally, and emotionally) are essential for everything that we do. We all have friends or relatives who have experienced life-altering challenges. They have been forever changed by the limitations placed on their body or mind by the illness. Do we place enough importance on the maintenance of our health? Are we willing to go the extra mile to do all that we can to ensure our health makes it to retirement with us?

Well-being should be a priority along with material growth. For the past three decades, the small Asian country of Bhutan has championed a new approach to development, which measures prosperity through gross national happiness and the spiritual, physical, social and environmental health of its citizens rather than by GDP (Gross Domestic Product). This approach is attracting a lot of interest.

It is NaturoMedic.com's desire to see a similar shift in thinking about health occur in our part of the world. Health can be a very controversial topic for a country or government. Take the United States, for example. It is likely that elections have been lost or won over the subject of health care. Little or no emphasis is placed on having a long-term health strategy by our mainstream medical system. And where the emphasis is put can make a world of difference…

HEALTH**NOW**HERE HEALTH**NOW**HERE

Are we suggesting that the current Canadian or American health care system should be discarded? Of course not. But we do need to recognize their limitations. When only the symptoms of a problem are addressed, a Band-Aid solution is provided and the root cause will never be cured. In North America, prescription drug trends have increased exponentially over the past 20 years. According to Statistics Canada in 2005, pharmacists dispensed on average 35 prescriptions per person aged 60 to 79 and 74 prescriptions per person aged 80 or older, with an overall average of **14 prescriptions per Canadian** citizen. In 2011, American doctors wrote 4.02 billion prescriptions, roughly equating to about 13 prescriptions for every man, woman and child. Society today places a lot of value on quick fixes and instant results – and we expect the same in the area of health. Unfortunately that kind of worldview does not lend itself to long-term strategies and results.

We need to be willing to invest in a health strategy that will target the root causes of our health concerns and commit to making the changes necessary to achieve our health goals. Similar health strategies have existed throughout the world. For instance, Traditional Chinese Medicine has continued to emphasize long-term health for over 5000 years. Homeopathy has existed for the past 200 years and has stressed the importance of disease prevention and treating the underlying factors. In North America, the first homeopathic hospital was opened in 1832. By the early 1900s, there were 22 homeopathic medical schools, 100 homeopathic hospitals and over 1,000 homeopathic pharmacies in the United States. Mortality (death) rates in homeopathic hospitals were often 50% to 88% less than those in medical hospitals. This well-established profession is commonly practiced especially in India. These two methods of medicine are examples that a health care system designed to conquer the root cause and prevent disease can exist. Moreover, it further demonstrates that this type of health strategy, which at one time was established in North America, has the potential for resurgence in our current medical system.

NaturoMedic.com approaches health from this angle. Our hope is that more and more people will come to recognize the need for greater continuity in our health care system. Instead of tearing down the existing health care structure, it is our aim to see it improved as we build on the many things it already has to offer.

Our desire is to see our patients taking steps to achieve optimal health in every area of their life. This includes the necessity of goal setting and an effective health strategy.

Assessing your current approach to health is essential to overcoming the obstacles to success. Establishing what you would like to achieve, setting high goals, embracing a proven strategy and developing methods of accountability are indispensable to your commitment and persistence. Being blessed with good health has now begun on your winding path through life. The lessons of the Health Navigator await.

--"Dream it. Plan it. Do it"--

References:

1. http://themedicalsanctuary.com.au/health/dopamine-and-reaching-our-goals/
2. http://michaelgholmes.com/why-goal-setters-change-the-world/
3. http://www.achieve-goal-setting-success.com/health-goals.html
4. http://toomuchonherplate.com/prioritize-yourself-and-be-more-effective-in-your-life
5. Locke, Edwin A.; Latham, Gary P. Building a practically useful theory of goal setting and task motivation: A 35-year odyssey. American Psychologist, Vol 57(9), Sep 2002, 705-717. http://faculty.washington.edu/janegf/goalsetting.html
6. Locke, Edwin A.; Shaw, Karyll N.; Saari, Lise M.; Latham, Gary P. Goal setting and task performance: 1969–1980.Psychological Bulletin, Vol 90(1), Jul 1981, 125-152. http://www.dtic.mil/dtic/tr/fulltext/u2/a086584.pdf
7. http://www.guardian.co.uk/world/2012/dec/01/bhutan-wealth-happiness-counts
8. http://www.homeopathyworldcommunity.com/profiles/blogs/who-declares-homoeopathy-as
9. http://www.dominican.edu/dominicannews/study-backs-up-strategies-for-achieving-goals

Chapter 2

NaturoMedic.com's Health Strategy

NaturoMedic.com's Health Strategy

My Health Navigator is a tool designed to inform and encourage readers about an effective health strategy that has been successfully implemented with thousands of patients over the past twenty years. As authors and as a clinic, our purpose is to direct and walk alongside our patients and readers as they seek to reach their health goals. Our strategy is designed to address the true nature of disease and promote an attainable definition of health.

The World Health Organization (WHO) has defined health as "a state of complete physical, mental and social well-being and not merely the absence of disease or infirmity." Despite no amendments to this statement since 1948, mainstream medicine continues to define health as the absence of disease. Like the WHO, NaturoMedic.com seeks not only to view health as the absence of disease, but also as a state of well-being in which disease causing factors are identified and addressed in every area of an individual's life. By striving for continual physical, emotional, spiritual and social optimization, we at NaturoMedic.com aspire to increase vitality to **Give Life to the Living™!**

Our strategy is to progress through **The Health Continuum™ in order to treat disease, treat functional disorders and prevent disease while progressing towards health optimization**. In order to accomplish this, improvements to health are made through successive therapeutic sessions to **increase quality of life, vitality and energy**. There are many disease causing factors which require identification and isolation in order to attain and maintain one's optimal well-being. At NaturoMedic.com, our health strategy includes 5 key principles.

1. The Health Continuum™:

Functional Disorder vs. Pathological Disease

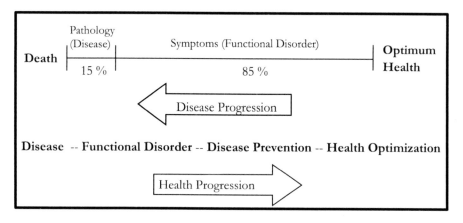

The first foundational principle of our strategy is The Health Continuum™ which illustrates the progression of disease. A visit to your medical doctor (MD) will usually begin with a symptom. In some cases, the MD may run multiple tests that do not present a diagnosis; their investigations come back within normal limits. There may be no signs of a pathological disease, but you still do not feel well. This may actually be due to a functional problem. In fact 85% of visits to MDs are for functional problems and not pathological ones. A functional disorder requires a tune up rather than significant intervention by your MD. In other words, you are not sick enough to qualify for treatment under the current system of healthcare. Therefore, you are left with symptoms without a long term strategy to successfully address them. Interestingly, Traditional Chinese Medicine functioned completely opposite to our system today. In ancient times, Chinese doctors were only paid as they maintained the health of their patients. If the patient became ill, the doctor was expected to provide free treatment. Their main goal was to promote optimal health and rectify functional disorders before pathology becomes established. As NDs our focus is to ultimately guide you through the Health Continuum™ by providing disease treatment, functional disorder treatment and disease prevention on the road to achieving optimal health.

2. The Health Cup Analogy™: Multifactorial vs. Monocausal

Another distinctive principle of our health strategy is that at NaturoMedic.com, we always look for the root cause of the problem. What are the factors causing poor health? There are usually several in a chronic condition (multifactorial) or there may be just one in an acute condition like an injury (monocasual). Modern pharmaceutical medicine prefers the monocausal disease philosophy as this promotes the idea of the magic bullet or miracle pill. One pill to address one symptom. Or one intervention to address one symptom. The Health Navigator proposes a different strategy. All possible factors are taken into consideration in order to properly assess and treat the cause of your health concerns. Humans are complicated beings. Over 1 trillion chemical reactions occurring in our bodies every second. Neurons fire every millisecond. We are very complex organisms indeed.

The Health Cup Analogy™: Imagine your body as a cup which represents your well-being. Your health cup is constantly being filled by various factors (these could include: pollution, diet, stress, microorganisms, etc.). Overall these burdens can be categorized into 5 main sections: Environment, Lifestyle, Body, Mind and Spirit see (Fig. 1).

Multiple factors accumulate as we progress through life and eventually your cup overflows resulting in functional symptoms or possibly disease. Most prescription medications regrettably do not address the causal problems. Instead they give you a larger cup to catch the overflow (Fig. 2). The symptoms are given temporary relief (the magic bullet or miracle drug) but the factors causing those symptoms are not eliminated. So the cup overflows again. This necessitates another stronger prescription (another miracle drug) to deal with an ever–expanding litany of symptoms, but not addressing the multitude of causes (Fig. 3). In order to obtain long-term health, we must treat the cause by identifying, isolating and/or altering the factors filling up your cup. Emptying your cup of these negative influences will lead to a true recovery rather than a suppression of symptoms.

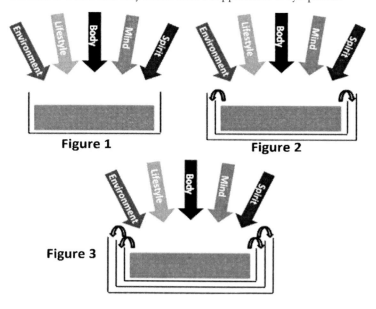

Figure 1

Figure 2

Figure 3

Pharmaceutical treatment of headaches is an excellent example of an immediate Band-Aid solution. Tylenol gives your symptoms relief by providing a bigger cup (Fig. 2), but it does not isolate any factors actually causing the headache. If causal factors, like diet, stress and environment are ignored then after a while, the Tylenol fails to work, forcing the need for a stronger medication. This creates a larger cup but none of the causal factors have been successfully treated. The cycle continues as the medications progress to Imitrex, then Cafergot, Fiorinal, nerve blocks or botox (Fig. 3). This provides symptomatic relief but the cause again is not addressed. Arthritis and heart disease are conditions which follow similar patterns.

- For arthritis, pain relief begins with Tylenol or Advil, followed by Non-Steroidal Anti-Inflammatories (Celebrex, Naproxen), then steroids, onto chemotherapeutic medications such as methotrexate and eventually joint replacement.

- For heart disease, various blood pressure medications are prescribed, followed by blood thinners and cholesterol lowering pills. Gradually increasing the number of prescriptions for each of the above while continuously monitoring for when to provide surgical intervention.

More prescriptions provide a larger cup, yet no one is isolating the factors filling up the cup and contributing to these disease conditions. Discovering the various causal factors is essential to eliminating disease and reaching your health goals.

Everyone is physiologically unique and the roadmap to health is dependent upon assessing the whole person. Modern medicine has isolated the body into different segments (i.e. dermatology, endocrinology, rheumatology, etc.), with each specialization acting independently of the other. At NaturoMedic.com, we acknowledge the complex interrelationships of environment, lifestyle, body, mind and spirit thus believing each segment works synergistically with the others. The person as a whole must be taken into account in order to create an effective plan to continue in the right direction on The Health Continuum™.

3. Healing Crisis vs. Disease Crisis

The third foundational principle in our health strategy is the well accepted naturopathic concept of a healing crisis. The path to health is not easy; you may feel temporarily worse before you get better. These may not be the encouraging words you wish to read although the change of symptoms is usually a positive sign. A healing crisis is associated with the emptying of your cup and removal of a disease causing factor. When the burden is isolated some symptoms initially become worse as the body now has more energy to focus on healing another area. This is what is commonly known as a **healing crisis**. Your energy and symptoms are the keys to determining whether this is a healing crisis or disease crisis. According to Constantine Hering, the father of American homeopathy, as healing progresses, symptoms appear in the reverse order of occurrence, from the top down, inside out and from the most vital to least vital organs. Therefore, if your energy is increasing while symptoms worsen or old ailments return, you are going through a healing crisis. In contrast, a **disease crisis**, is when the overall progression of symptoms, energy and disease continue to worsen. The experience of a healing crisis, while not initially enjoyable, can often be accompanied by a sensation of euphoria as the burden in the cup is being eliminated. Do not let a healing crisis discourage you. Stay focused and remember your ultimate goal.

4. The Weakest Link™

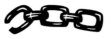 The fourth of our five health strategy principles is the importance of supporting The Weakest Link™. To reiterate, at NaturoMedic.com we acknowledge the complex interrelationships of the environment, lifestyle, body, mind and spirit. The various physiological functions and processes of your body can be represented by an intricate chain. Each link represents a different organ, hormone, muscle, neurotransmitter, enzyme, protein, etc. The strength of the chain is dependent upon the connection of each link. In regards to health, the common expression "a chain is only as strong as its weakest link" holds true. When one area is not functioning properly, the body attempts to compensate for the weakness. At NaturoMedic.com, we begin the health journey by systematically isolating disease causing factors and supporting the most fragile link to help rebuild your system. By strengthening The Weakest Link™, the whole chain becomes stronger, resolving many symptoms without the need for further intervention. The body has the ability to heal itself is given the right conditions and support. *Vis Medicatrix Naturae* is the latin phrase that refers to the healing power of nature. It is one of the founding beliefs of Naturopathic Medicine. It is our essential life energy (*Qi*, vital force) that helps us to heal and maintain balance. By identifying obstacles and reinforcing areas of weakness, we are fostering the power of the *vis* to promote healing as your cup is purged. There are many layers to health. On your journey, each layer must be successfully peeled away, like an onion, to reach your optimal health.

5. Docere (Doctor as Teacher)

The final key principle of NaturoMedic.com's health strategy is the naturopathic concept of doctor as teacher. Education is critical to treating disease and progressing toward the achievement of optimal health. A Naturopathic Doctor (ND) plays a very crucial role in this process; an ND acts as a teacher. Disease can manifest in a variety of forms, but by understanding the factors that contribute to the problem and how they can be corrected, health is attainable. The knowledge contained in the Health Navigator will empower and motivate you to make informed decisions and take control of your health.

What to Expect

NaturoMedic.com's health strategy incorporates these 5 key principles as well as methods of accountability to ensure commitment and goal attainment. Obtaining a full health history is essential for identifying obstacles and individualizing your strategy. There are health practitioners whose strategy is to give supplements that address every issue at once. You will feel better, but unfortunately you will always be dependent upon the supplements or the practitioner to maintain your health.

At NaturoMedic.com we take a systematic approach. By isolating factors in a sequential way and supporting The Weakest Link™, we can provide minimal supplementation, save you money and help you take control of your own health. The education about disease causing factors is invaluable to your success. When you learn how disease progresses, you can actively work towards disease prevention and the optimization of your health.

It is necessary to understand that your present state of health may be the result of an entire lifetime. Therefore to expect an overnight cure is unrealistic. Healing is a process that takes time and commitment. At NaturoMedic.com, we do not chase symptoms. We seek to find the root of the problem and address it. To achieve this we want to know all about you!

To assist you in getting the most out of your doctor visits and attaining your health goals, we have created tools to help you track your progress on a routine basis. The **Symptom Tracker™** and **Lab Tracker™** are designed to keep you in tune with your body, allowing you to see the long-term change in your concerns and motivating you to fulfill your goals. The **Pill Minder™** is a great addition for maintaining your treatment schedule. Knowing when to administer medications and observing the effects on symptoms can significantly amplify your progress. By utilizing these tools you will be able to monitor your health progress over time. This will boost your self-confidence and provide the impetus to push forward to your goal of disease prevention and health optimization. These handy tools are currently available in hard copy form at NaturoMedic.com.

At NaturoMedic.com our goal is to work with you to provide education, service and access to effective healing therapies geared towards giving you the health results you desire. In order to be successful, your cooperation as a member of your own health team is essential. All the necessary forms, tools and products are available, however without your participation it will be difficult to achieve the results you desire. This is equivalent to asking us to wrestle a disease to the ground with one arm tied behind our backs.

Before entering into an effective treatment relationship, NaturoMedic.com will propose a **Health Commitment™**. The NaturoMedic.com team is determined to provide safe, effective, individualized treatment that addresses your concerns and is intended to provide disease prevention while working towards optimal health. NaturoMedic.com will strive to reach these goals throughout your treatment program. If at any time you feel we are not doing our part, please provide us with your feedback immediately.

The opportunity of having a guide with an effective strategy for achieving your goals will accelerate your journey to health. The following chapters will share in depth some potential obstacles and therapeutic possibilities. **Part I** of the book will continue to identify in greater detail the various factors in our life that influence our level of health. **Part II** will outline some of the treatments that may be provided by our Naturopathic Doctors.

References:
1. http://www.who.int/about/definition/en/print.html
2. Kroenke, K., & A.D.Mangelsdorff. Common Symptoms in Ambulatory Care: Incidence, Evaluation, Therapy & Outcome. American Journal of Medicine 86:262-266, 1989. http://www.amjmed.com/article/0002-9343(89)90293-3/abstract
3. http://www.acupuncture.com/Conditions/pulse_prevent.htm
4. http://www.homeoint.org/biograph/heringen.htm

Chapter 3

Disease Causing Factors: Environment

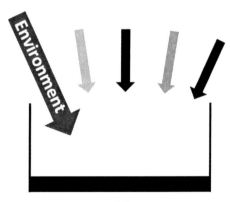

Air Quality

Just what am I breathing?

Indoor Air in the Home

The greatest personal exposure to volatile organic compounds (VOCs) is from air in our homes and not from the outdoors. The US Environmental Protection Agency released a study in 1985, the Total Exposure Assessment Methodology (TEAM), which revealed very high exposure of 11 VOCs in personal respired air. The TEAM study was consistent with earlier results. Higher levels of one or more VOCs can be found indoors and are often 10 times higher than the outdoors.

The elevated levels of compounds in household air can be attributed to industrial advances. In the 1970s, building techniques were changed to accommodate for the "oil shortage". New energy-efficient homes that would reduce air exchange between inside and outside in order to decrease the amount of energy needed to maintain the climate were emphasized. Unfortunately, the newer homes would also retain the gas venting from construction materials (known as off-gassing) at higher levels than older homes. During the same timeframe, a tremendous increase in VOC containing compounds was introduced in building materials, fabrics and home furnishings. Whether outdoors or indoors, at work or at home, the truth is, solvents are being inhaled. The most concerning areas are often the workplace and the home.

Carpet as a Major Source of Indoor Air Chemicals

Carpeting alone can be a significant factor in the emission of VOCs and retention of pesticide residues. Anderson Labs began testing carpet samples for its effect on the immune system. In testing over 400 samples, they found neurotoxins present in more than 90% of samples, including some that can cause death. In 1993, the EPA sponsored the Non-Occupational Pesticide Exposure Study (NOPES) which confirmed that indoor air is indeed more toxic than outdoor air. The EPA researchers found that concentrations of pesticides in indoor air were highest in the summer and lowest in the winter, corresponding with the seasonal patterns of pesticide use. A partial list of the frequently found chemicals and pesticides are included in the following tables.

A partial list of chemicals present in carpet

Formaldehyde	Azulene	Phthalic acid esters
TCE	Benzene	Xylene
Acetonitrite	Methyl	Methacrylic acid
1-Ethyl-3-	methacrylate	1-Chloronaphthalene
methylbenzene	Styrene	1,2,3-Trimethylbenzene
1,2,4-	Ethylzylene	1-Methyl-3-Propylbenzene
Trimethylbenzene	Biphenyl	Cyclopentadiene-ethenyl-2-
4-Phenylcylohexane	Isocyanates	ethylene
2-Butyloctanol-1	Dipehyl ether	Undecane, 2,6-Dimethyl
1,3,5-Cycloheptatriene	Butadiene	1,4-Dihydroxyacenophthene
Dodecane	Hexadecanol	Hexamethylene Triamine
1-Methylnapthlalaene	1-H-indene	2-Methylnapthalene
1-Methyl-4-Tridecen	Polyzcrylates	5-Methyltridecane
Octadecenyl Amine	Oxarium	Tetradecene
2,3,7-Trimethldecane		

Thrasher J, Broughton A. The Poisoning of Our Homes and Workplaces.
Santa Ana, CA: Seadora, Inc. Publ; 1989

Pesticides Detected Most Frequently in Carpet Dust in NOPES Study

Heptachlor	DDT
Chlorpyrifos	ortho-Phenylphenol
Aldrin	Propoxur
Dieldrin	Diazinon
Chlordane	Carbaryl
Atrazine	

Whitemore RW, Immerman FW, Camann DE, et al. Non-occupational
exposures to pesticides for residents of two U.S. cities. Arch Environ Contam
Toxicol 1994; 26:47-59.

Toddlers and infants are at greatest risk for exposure to carpet and dust bonded pesticides as they spend the most time in contact with carpet and are continuously placing things from the carpet into their mouths. According to the NOPES study, this route of exposure likely provides infants and toddlers with nearly all of non-dietary exposure to certain solvents: DDT, aldrin, altrazine, and carbaryl.

Adverse Health Effects of Solvents

The U.S. Environmental Protection Agency performed the National Human Adipose Tissue survey that identified 4 solvents which were present in 100% of participants tissue samples tested across the country (xylene, dichlorobenzene, ethylphenol, and styrene). Regular exposure of citizens to VOCs must have occurred over time in order for these solvents to be deposited in fat tissue.

VOCs act as both peripheral and central nervous system neurotoxins which can lead to diminished cognitive function and motor movements, tremors, decreased memory and reaction time, mood disorders, irritability and fatigue. Kidney damage, immunotoxicity and cancer have also been implicated.

Solvents have been found to affect hormone levels including decreased testosterone and increased insulin levels. As a result infertility, decreased sperm count, increased rates of spontaneous abortion and increased rates of fetal malformation have frequently manifested. Blood disorders have also been found to occur.

The indoor air levels of solvents and formaldehyde are closely associated with increased rates of asthma and chronic bronchitis especially in children. The typical presentation of low dose formaldehyde exposure includes upper respiratory irritations such as rhinitis, sinusitis and pharyngitis, lower respiratory symptoms of wheezing and persistent flu-like symptoms.

The quality of air in our home can have a direct impact on our health. The high levels of VOCs that have been found and their adverse effects are concerning, especially for children. Purifying the air we breathe and removing these solvents from our bodies is an important step in maintaining our overall well-being. For more information refer to the Toxic Home to see your daily exposure (www.everydayexposures.com)

References:
1. Environmental Medicine Part 2 - Health Effects of and Protection from Ubiquitous Airborne Solvent Exposures Walter J. Crinnion, ND
2. Toxic Nation Report (A Report on pollution in Canadians) 2005
3. Chemical Canada (Toxic Nation Report)
4. Thrasher J, Broughton A. The Poisoning of Our Homes and Workplaces. Santa Ana, CA: Seadora, Inc. Publ; 1989
5. Whitemore RW, Immerman FW, Camann DE, et al. Non-occupational exposures to pesticides for residents of two U.S. cities. Arch Environ Contam Toxicol 1994; 26:47-59.
6. Wallace LA, Pellizzari ED, Hartwell TD, et al. Personal exposure, indoor-outdoor relationships, and breath levels of toxic air pollutants measured for 355 persons in New Jersey. EPA 0589
7. Wallace LA, Pellizzari ED, Hartwell TD, et al. Personal exposure, indoor-outdoor relationships, and breath levels of toxic air pollutants measured for 425 persons in urban, suburban and rural areas. EPA 0589. Presented at annual meeting of Air Pollution Control Association, June 25, 1984. San Francisco, CA.

Environmental Allergies

Sneeze, Swell, and Swipe

 Allergies are a common problem affecting approximately 30% of the population in North America. Environmental allergies can be caused by many factors including dust, mildew, mold spores, feathers, ragweed, tree pollen, flower pollen and even animal dander. Dust and mold allergies can occur all year round and not just during certain seasons. Exposure to these substances occurs daily while you are at home, at school, in the workplace or on your daily commute. Once the allergen is inhaled, your body responds by alerting the immune system and mounting an attack against it. First, the body produces an antibody to fight the allergen. The body perceives the allergen as a foreign invader, reacting in a similar manner to a virus or bacteria. The antibody attaches to mast cells (cells important in allergies) that are very abundant in the respiratory and digestive tracts. The mast cells explode, releasing histamine, the culprit responsible for the itchiness and runny nose.

Allergy symptoms can be categorized into three levels of severity. Mild reactions include congestion, sneezing, itchy or watery eyes. Moderate reactions may consist of breathing difficulties or itchiness on more than one area of the body. Anaphylaxis is a severe, life-threatening reaction that is rare. It may begin as a mild reaction, but within minutes progresses to swelling of the respiratory tract, difficulties breathing and swallowing, vomiting and diarrhea, etc. Nut and bee allergies are familiar examples of anaphylaxis. Environmental allergies have more subtle effects on the body. With chronic exposure to these substances, low-level inflammation to the airway is not as obvious. Possible manifestations of chronic inflammation can include a tendency to have long-lasting colds, recurrent ear or sinus infections and coughing or wheezing after vigorous activities or with infections (asthma).

The current state of the body may also increase susceptibility to environmental allergens. The immune system is heavily dependent on proper digestion for the absorption of essential nutrients. The mucosal tissue that protects the digestive and respiratory system requires Vitamin A to function properly. Improper digestion can decrease absorption of Vitamin A and make the immune system more susceptible to environmental allergens. In addition the decreased strength of these tissues in the digestive tract further inhibits its function leading to a condition called 'leaky gut'—absorption of unnecessary particles that may trigger allergic reactions. For example, certain food allergens can resemble and act similar to environmental pollens and spores. Therefore during allergy season, the body being already sensitive to the food allergen reacts with the environmental allergen (a concept known as cross-reactivity). Cross reactivity can be caused by food additives, chemicals and artificial products. A strong digestive system would normally eliminate these from our body, however when the system is weakened, these substances can be absorbed and cause havoc. Maintaining a strong digestive system and immune system is important in reducing environmental triggers.

Depending on the allergy, the weather plays a significant role in the amount of allergen present in the environment. Wind increases transportation of allergens. Rain and dampness take pollens out of the air giving short-term relief but also encouraging the growth of certain fungal and mold spores. Hot and humid conditions influence the growth of a variety of allergenic spores. There are thousands of different types of spores present in the air throughout the year and many have seasonal variation. Knowing when these counts are elevated may help to prepare you for days that will create the most symptoms and may also help reduce your exposure. The weather network offers a seasonal pollen forecast, which provides counts for the common tree pollen and spores that occur from March to October. Please refer to http://www.theweathernetwork.com/pollenfx/canpollen_en to see the seasonal variation for your area. For US counts refer to http://www.weather.com/maps/activity/allergies/index_large.html.

References:
1. http://www.naturesintentionsnaturopathy.com/allergies/environmental-allergies.htm
2. http://www.parentscanada.com/baby/health/children-and-allergies.aspx
3. http://the-health-pages.com/topics/topics/education/environmental_allergies.html
4. http://www.theweathernetwork.com/index.php?product=pollenfx&pagecontent=background

Water Quality

I drank what?

 Water is essential to the body. The human body is roughly composed of 25% solid matter and 75% water. The brain alone consists of 85% water and blood is primarily 90% water. Water is necessary for survival and optimum function. The quality of water used to replenish the body is also significant.

Water and Heart Disease

The ability of water to affect cardiovascular health may not be a familiar topic. This well-studied relationship is dependent on two factors; hardness of water and the amount of total dissolved solids (TDS) in water. Hardness refers to the concentration of calcium and magnesium in the water supply whereas TDS measures all the minerals in drinking water, including calcium, magnesium, zinc, copper, chromium, selenium, etc. These two factors have been associated with lower mortality and heart disease. The Relationship of Water to the Risk of Dying study found that people who drank water higher in TDS had lower death rates from heart disease, cancer and chronic diseases than those who consumed water with lower amounts of TDS. Numerous major studies have analyzed drinking water since 1960 and each has concluded that areas with hard water had lower mortality rates from heart disease than areas with soft water. In fact, the National Academy of Sciences concluded that "an optimum conditioning of drinking water could reduce the amount of cardiovascular disease by as much as 15%".

Modern water softening techniques can also contribute to the problem. During the process, sodium is usually added to the water, replacing significant amounts of calcium and magnesium. The elevated level of sodium in the drinking water has an effect on blood pressure, contributing to hypertension and increased risk of developing heart disease.

Water and Cancer

The hardness of drinking water and the amount of TDS have been associated with cancer. The pH and the amount of contamination appear to play an influential role. Over 2100 organic and inorganic contaminants have been identified in U.S. drinking water since 1974. A 10-25% reduction in cancer deaths were found if the drinking water contained moderate levels of TDS, if the water was hard and if the water was alkaline (above 7.0). Alkaline water will not leech heavy metals or chemicals from pipes, decreasing the amount of harmful contaminates in our drinking water. The majority of water studies have concluded that drinking hard water with 300mg/L of TDS and an alkaline pH will reduce the risk of cancer mortality.

Fluorinated water has had a direct role in cancer related deaths. The National Cancer Institute stated in the Journal of Toxicology and Environmental Health (1977) that "more people have died in the last thirty years from cancer connected with fluoridation than all military deaths in the entire history of the United States". Genetic damage in plants, animals and birth defects in humans has been linked to toxicity from fluoride. Additional symptoms ranging from fatigue, headaches, urinary tract infections, diarrhea and allergic reactions have resulted with fluoride accumulation in the body. The National Research Council of Canada documented in an Environmental Fluoride study, the mutagenic effects of fluoride and the interference it has on the metabolism of calcium, magnesium and vitamin C. Fluoride was originally added to the drinking water to prevent tooth decay, however these adverse effects were not taken into consideration. One very interesting fact regarding tooth decay is that no genuine scientific research supports the belief that up to 1mg/L will prevent tooth decay. Dr. John Yiamouyiannis revealed in his book Fluoride: the Aging Factor, a court testimonial from Illinois whereby "the United States Center for Disease Control and the British Ministry of Health admit that no laboratory experiment has ever shown that one ppm (1mg/L) fluoride in the drinking water is effective in reducing tooth decay…" Judge Ronal A. Newman ruled that "a conclusion that fluoride is a safe and effective means of promoting dental health cannot be supported by this record." Then why is the addition of fluoride to our drinking water still advocated? New Zealand and the US found no difference in decay rates of permanent teeth at any age with fluorinated water. In fact, many countries including Germany, Spain, France and Sweden have discontinued the use of fluoride in their drinking water for health and legal reasons over the past thirty years. The long-term health effects of fluoridation should be taken into consideration. You can check with your local municipality to see if fluoride is still used in your area.

Chlorine is another chemical that demonstrates alarming concern in regards to cancer. Chlorine was added to the drinking water in the late 1890's and widely used in North America by 1920. In the chlorination process, chlorine combines with natural organic matter and decaying vegetation to create potent cancer causing substances. These carcinogens by law are not allowed to exceed 100 ppb (parts per billion), however many water systems surpass this limit. Studies completed in 1975 found that the number of chemical contaminants found in drinking water were actually closer to 300 ppb. According to the report, Trouble Waters on Tap, over 2100 contaminants have been detected in US drinking water since 1974; of which 190 are contaminants suspected to cause adverse effects, 97 are carcinogens, 82 are mutagens, 28 are toxic contaminants and 23 are tumour promoting agents. While the addition of chlorine was intended to improve the quality of our drinking water the amount of unhealthy substances produced in the process may actually be increasing the risk of developing cancer.

Chlorine and fluorine belong to the halide family on Chemistry's Periodic Table of Elements. These can displace another halide, iodine, in the body. Excess absorption of these can easily decrease the amount of iodine in the body contributing to high rates of thyroid disorders and cancer of the breast, ovary and prostate.

In summary, there are many factors to consider regarding the quality of the water we consume every day. The solution is not to abstain from drinking water as it is vitally essential to the human body. The idea is to drink soft water with high TDS, high pH, low amounts of fluorine, chlorine and other contaminants.

References:
1. Burk D. Fluoridation: A Burning Controversy. Bestways, April, 1982: 40-44
2. Burton AC, Comhill F. Correlation of Cancer Death Rates with Altitude and with the Quality of Water Supply of 100 Largest Cities in the United States. Journal Toxicology and Environmental Health 1977;3:465-478
3. Conacher D. Trouble Waters on Tap: Organic Chemicals in Public Drinking Water Systems and the Failure of Regulation. Wash., D.C.: Center for Study of Responsive Law, 1988: 114
4. Maugh TH. New Study Links Chlorination and Cancer. Science 1983; 211 (February 13):694.
5. National Research Council. Drinking Water and Health. Vol1:477. Wash.
6. Wilkins JR, Reiches NA, Kruse CW. Organic Chemical Contaminants in Drinking Water and Cancer. Am J. Epidemology 1979; 14:178-190
7. Yiamouyiannis JA. Fluoride: The Aging Factor. Delaware, OH: Health Action Press, 1983

Chemicals and Solvents

How polluted are you?

It is no longer a question of **if** you are exposed to chemicals but rather of **how much** exposure you have had? According to Dr. Rick Smith, executive director of Environmental Defense Canada, a Toronto-based environmental health group, "We are all polluted, it does not matter where you live, how old you are, how clean you live, if you eat organic food or if you get a lot of exercise. We all carry inside of us hundreds of different pollutants and these toxins are accumulating inside our bodies every day."

Chemical compounds present in our food, air and water are now found in every living being. The bioaccumulation of these compounds can cause a variety of health issues by negatively impacting the immune, neurological and hormonal systems. Toxicity in these systems can lead to immune dysfunction, autoimmune diseases, asthma, allergies, cancers, cognitive deficit, mood changes, neurological illnesses, changes in libido, reproductive dysfunction and glucose dysregulation.

Our health can be greatly affected by the environment, therefore it is important to understand what we are exposed to. Since 1976, the US Environmental Protection Agency has been collecting and analyzing samples of fat tissue from thousands of participants for the presence of toxic compounds. In 1982, this nationwide annual program, National Human Adipose Tissue Survey (NHATS), looked for 54 different environmental chemical toxins. In 100% of samples, 9 chemicals were found, another 9 toxins were in 91-98% of samples and a total of 20 compounds were found in 76% of individual specimens. These chemicals were either carcinogens or neurotoxins that included DDT (DDE/DDD), PCBs and Xylene.

In Canada, a similar cocktail of chemicals was detected by a Report on Pollution in Canadians from the non-profit group Environmental Defense. The Toxic Nation study conducted by Environmental Defense was the first in Canada to test for a broad range of chemicals in the average Canadian across the country. The results detected 60 of the 88 chemicals in 11 volunteers: these included 18 heavy metals, 5 PBDEs, 14 PCBs, 1 perfluorinated chemical, 10 organochlorine pesticides, 5 organophosphate insecticide metabolites and seven VOCs (volatile organic compounds). On average, 44 chemicals were detected in each volunteer; examples ranged from 41 carcinogens, 27 hormone disruptors, 21 respiratory toxins and 53 reproductive/developmental toxins. These high amounts of chemicals in our bodies are concerning.

A National Report by Environmental Defense and the Canadian Environmental Law Association showed that the volume of chemicals released in Canada increased by 49% between 1995 and 2002. In 2003, air pollution emitted by Canadian industries alone totaled over 4.1 billion kilograms (Table 1). Exposure to these toxic chemicals has been linked to many ailments that have been increasing in Canadians in recent decades. These include several forms of cancer, reproductive disorders, birth defects, asthma and neurodevelopment disorders.

Table 1. Pollutant releases by industry in Canada in 2003.

Substance Type	Amount Released
Carcinogens	Nearly 18 million kg
Hormone disruptors	Over 14 million kg
Respiratory Toxins	Over 4.3 billion kg
Reproductive/developmental toxins	Over 1 billion kg

Source: PollutionWatch analysis of data from the National Pollutant Release Inventory, Environment Canada (October, 2005).

Environmental Defence. (2005, October 15). Pollution Watch Compilation: Create a Pollution Report. Available at http://www.pollutionwatch.org

The pollution in Canadians extends all the way to Ottawa. Four federal politicians volunteered to be tested for over 100 different chemicals. Of the 103 chemicals, 61 were detected in the four participants, Rona Ambrose (the Minister of the Environment), Tony Clement (the Minister of Health), the late Jack Layton (Leader of the NDP) and John Godfrey (Liberal Environment Critic). Many of the chemicals detected are associated with adverse health effects (Table 2).

Table 2: Number of chemicals detected in the politicians that are linked to a listed known or suspected health effect.

Chemicals Effect on Health	Total Detected	Number of Chemicals Detected that are Linked to a Listed Known or Suspected Health Effect			
		Jack Layton	Rona Ambrose	Tony Clement	John Godfrey
Carcinogen	54	45	42	47	47
Hormone Disrupter	37	34	35	37	37
Respiratory Toxin	16	11	8	9	9
Reproductive/Developmental Toxin	54	45	42	47	47
Neurotoxin	33	29	29	33	33
No data on Health Effects	3	3	2	2	2

*See Appendix 3 for information on how chemicals were categorized accordidng to known or suspected health effects.

Toxic Nation: ON PARLIAMENT HILL A
Report on Pollution in Four Canadian Politicians

These were not the only polluted politicians. The most recent Toxic Body Burden study tested Ontario politicians including, Premier Dalton McGuinty, NDP

Leader Howard Hampton and the Progressive Conservative Leader John Tory for 70 different chemicals. In the three volunteers, 46 toxins were detected and many are linked to negative health effects including 33 carcinogens, 24 hormone disruptors, 9 respiratory toxins, 39 reproductive/developmental toxins and 12 neurotoxins.

Internationally, Canada has one of the worst pollution records among industrialized countries. From emissions of air pollutants, like VOCs and sulphur oxides, to the production of nuclear waste, Canada consistently ranks at the bottom of the 30 industrialized countries that report to the Environmental Data Compendium of the Organization for Economic Co-operation and Development (OECD). Canada has held on to its poor environmental ranking for over a decade, now placing 28th out of 30 countries in 1992, 2002 and again in 2005.

Adverse Health Effects of Solvents

There is much evidence connecting these chemical compounds to health, however how much effect can they have on the body?

VOCs (volatile organic compounds) act as both peripheral and central nervous system neurotoxins. They can cause diminished cognitive function and motor movements, decreased memory and reaction time, mood disorders, irritability and fatigue. Kidney damage, immunotoxicity and cancer have also been implicated.

Solvents have been found to affect hormone levels, including decreased testosteroe and increased insulin levels. Infertility, decreased sperm count, increased rates of spontaneous abortion and increased rates of fetal malformation have resulted. Blood disorders have also been found to occur.

In the last 50 years, the global production and use of manufactured chemicals increased substantially. More than 80,000 new chemicals have been created and the quantity of chemicals produced, used and released into the environment is drastically higher now than a generation ago. Studies have found toxic chemicals in every corner of every country-in the land, the air, the water, wildlife, people's blood and women's breast milk. It is clear that the environment we live in contains many pollutants. These chemicals can be found in every individual and the implications are very concerning. Removing these compounds from the body and decreasing our body burden of toxins is important to our overall health.

References:

1. Environmental Medicine, Part 1: The Human Burden of Environmental Toxins and Their Common Health Effects. Walter J. Crinnion, ND , Alt Med Rev. Vol 5, No 1, 2000.
2. Toxic Nation: ON PARLIAMENT HILL A Report on Pollution in Four Canadian Politicians
3. Toxic Nation: At Queen's Park A Report on Pollution in Three Ontario Politicians
4. The CDC Fourth National Report on Human Exposure to Environmental Chemicals: What it Tells Us About our Toxic Burden and How it Assists Environmental Medicine Physicians Walter J.Crinnion
5. André Picard, The Globe and Mail - Wednesday, November 09, 2005
6. Toxic Nation Report (A Report on pollution in Canadians) 2005
7. Environmental Defence. (2005, October 15). PollutionWatch Compilation: Create a Pollution Report. Available at http://www.pollutionwatch.org

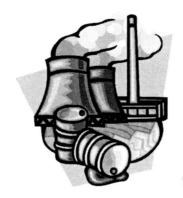

Pesticides

Who is the target?

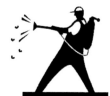

Pesticides are primarily used in agriculture to protect crops and livestock. They consist of insecticides, herbicides and fungicides designed to prevent, destroy and repel pests. The killing of primary pests with pesticides has paved the way for secondary pests to come to the forefront. Since 1945 overall pesticide use has risen 3,300%, while overall crop loss due to insects has risen only 20%. Of the 2.5 million tons of pesticides used worldwide each year, **less than 0.1 % reaches the target pest**. In other words, 99% of the applied pesticides are not achieving their goal and are being released into the environment. Many will persist for years and travel far from the area of application, exposing humans to these harmful substances.

Residues of pesticides remain in or on the treated food we consume. Drinking water can be contaminated as runoff or leaching can occur through the soil and persist for decades. The use of pesticides on lawns, gardens and ornamental plants can often lead to exposure in the home. Personal insect repellants and flea and tick products on pets are also sources of exposure. As a bystander, you can easily be exposed to these products in public areas such as schools, parks and recreational areas.

The toxicity and the amount of pesticides a person are exposed to can have a direct influence on their health. For instance, a pesticide with a low toxicity and high exposure may cause similar risks as a pesticide with higher toxicity and low exposure. The accumulated exposure to multiple substances can have greater impact than their individual effects. The damage to the body could increase exponentially for each pesticide we come in contact with. The health effect of most pesticides has been assessed yet the combination of these products is far from being fully understood.

The health and safety of pesticides can greatly depend on the type of pesticide. Some of the main pesticides include:

Organophosphates: a group of insecticides used in both agricultural and non-agricultural sites. They were originally developed in the early 19th century and some were used as chemical weapons (nerve agents) in World War II. These pesticides disrupt an important enzyme responsible for regulating a critical neurotransmitter in the body, acetylcholine, which can lead to damaging effects on the nervous system. Several of these pesticides have been discontinued and restricted in residential use.

Carbamate: a group of pesticides used in homes, gardens and agriculture. They can affect the function of acetylcholine by disrupting an enzyme responsible for its regulation. The enzyme effects are usually reversible.

Organochlorine: an insecticide commonly used in the past. Many have been removed from the market due to their damaging effects on health and their persistence in environment (e.g. DDT and chlordane). Soil-based DDT is incorporated into grasses growing in the soil, into cattle consuming the grass and eventually into the milk and fat tissue of cows. The half-life of DDT ranges between 4-30 years.

Pyrethroid: pesticides developed as a synthetic version of the naturally occurring pesticide found in chrysanthemums, known as pyrethrin. They have been modified to increase their stability in the environment. Some synthetic pyrethroids are toxic to the nervous system.

Arsenic based pesticides: discontinued in the U.S. but still widely available in certain countries. Homes and farmers have leftover supplies that remain to be a risk. Arsenic has life-threatening effects in the body specifically to the central nervous system, blood vessels, kidney and liver.

Mercury based fungicides: mainly used as seed protectants. Many mercury compounds have been prohibited for several years. Among the most toxic pesticides ever developed. Severe and often fatal neurological disease have occurred when mercury-treated grains have been consumed directly or through the meat of animals fed mercury-treated seeds.

Pesticides can have a variety of effects especially on the nervous system. Some pesticides may be carcinogens, while others may affect hormones and the endocrine system in the body. One important factor in uptake and storage of chemicals is whether they are water or fat soluble. Water soluble compounds have a low potential for bioaccumulation as they do not easily enter cells. Fat loving chemicals pass more easily into the body's cells through the cell membrane where they can accumulate in fatty tissues. Fat soluble compounds do not need to be re-sprayed following a rainfall as opposed to water soluble. The National Human Adipose Tissue Survey identified multiple pesticides stored in human fat tissue (*please refer to Chemicals and Solvents for more information*). Numerous studies have also shown persistent levels of chlorinated pesticide residues, including DDT, in breast milk that correlated directly with the level in maternal adipose tissue. In the body, when detoxification pathways are working efficiently, we can effectively deal with some exposure to pesticides. With increased exposure, the body removes the toxin from the blood, but stores the chemical in fat; therefore when fat reserves are called upon to provide energy, the chemical is remobilized and released back into the bloodstream leading to toxic effects. The negative impact pesticides can have in our body is alarming.

Food can often be a large source of contamination. The Environment Working Group (EWG) offers a Shopper's Guide to Pesticides in Produce that determines which fruits and vegetables have the most pesticide residues (please refer to www.ewg.org for more information). Produce with a thin skin are more susceptible to contamination through absorption of the pesticide.

12 Most Contaminated Produce Items

1. Peaches
2. Apples
3. Sweet Bell Peppers
4. Celery
5. Nectarines
6. Strawberries
7. Cherries
8. Pears
9. Grapes (Imported)
10. Spinach
11. Lettuce
12. Potatoes

12 Least Contaminated Produce Items

1. Onions
2. Avocado
3. Sweet Corn (Frozen)
4. Pineapples
5. Mango
6. Asparagus
7. Sweet Peas (Frozen)
8. Kiwi Fruit
9. Bananas
10. Cabbage
11. Broccoli
12. Papaya

Another tool is the Interactive Toxic Home. An excellent and fun resource to see the common toxins that are present in different areas and rooms in the home (you can access the interactive site at www.everydayexposures.com). With the many possible sources of pesticides in our environment, it is important to stay informed and try to limit your exposure.

References:
1. http://www.hc-sc.gc.ca/ewh-semt/pubs/contaminants/pesticides-eng.php
2. http://www.epa.gov/pesticides/
3. www.ewg.org
4. www.everydayexposures.com
5. Crinnion, W. Environmental Medicine, Part 4: Pesticides – Biologically Persistent and Ubiquitous Toxin
6. Routt Reigart, J & Roberts J.R. Recognition and Management of Pesticide Poisonings. 5th edit. 1999. United States Environmental Protection Agency. United Book Press, Baltimore, MD.

Heavy Metals
Individually toxic, synergistically lethal

 In the past 30 years, the growing concern for a reduction in environmental pollution has led to continuing research on the toxic effects of heavy metals. Mankind's exposure to heavy metals is not new to our environment; in fact, we have repeatedly been poisoning ourselves throughout history. In the late Roman Empire, aristocrats used to drink out of lead cups and many water lines were made out of lead pipes. Several hundred years passed before a connection between mental illness and contaminated drinking water was established. The use of mercury for the treatment of acute and chronic infection was used in the 1700s. Decades passed before the neurotoxic and immunosuppressive effects of mercury were documented.

Virtually all metals can produce toxicity when ingested in sufficient quantities. Most metals have a very narrow therapeutic margin before they become neurotoxic and in some cases carcinogenic. The common heavy metals include: arsenic, lead, mercury, cadmium, aluminum, iron, copper, nickel, silver and beryllium.

Everyone is exposed to heavy metals in our environment and therefore we all have certain levels inside our bodies. The accumulation of this exposure has negative impacts on our health.

Heavy Metals and Health Effects

Chemicals and heavy metals are ranked by the US Agency for Toxic Substances & Disease Registry (ATDSR) based on frequency, toxicity and the potential for human exposure. Only 250 substances are considered to be on the ATDSR list of 847 candidate substances.

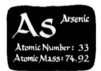

As Arsenic

Atomic Number: 33
Atomic Mass: 74.92

Arsenic: Ranked #1 on ATSDR Priority List of Hazardous Substances (2011)

- May be exposed to arsenic in the air, drinking water and food (usually the largest source)
- Prior to 2003, arsenic was used in the production of wood preservatives, primarily copper chromated arsenate (CCA)
  - ➤ Sawing, sanding or burning wood can generate arsenic contaminated sawdust or smoke
- Various organic arsenicals are used as herbicides, pesticides for ants, termites and spiders and antimicrobial additives for animal and poultry feed

- **Health Effects**
  - ➤ Inhalation of inorganic arsenic may cause respiratory irritation, nausea, skin effects and increased risk of lung cancer
  - ➤ Long term oral exposure to low levels of inorganic arsenic may cause dermal effects (such as hyperpigmentation and hyperkeratosis, corns and warts) and peripheral neuropathy characterized by a numbness in the hands and feet that may progress to a painful "pins and needles" sensation. There may also be an increased risk of skin cancer, bladder cancer and lung cancer.

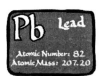

Lead: Ranked #2 on ATSDR Priority List of Hazardous Substances (2011)

Atomic Number: 82
Atomic Mass: 207.20

- Prior to 1991, lead was found in gasoline, paint and plumbing fixtures and therefore could easily accumulate in the body. Lead can remain in the body for a min of 30 years.
- The most likely source of exposure is ingestion of contaminated food and drinking water
  - ➤ Exposure can also occur via inadvertent ingestion of contaminated soil/dust or lead-based paint
  - ➤ Lead can leach into drinking water from lead-soldered joints or leaded pipes
  - ➤ Some types of hair dyes and cosmetics (lipsticks) may contain lead compounds
  - ➤ Other potential sources of exposure are hobbies that use lead: fishing weights, soldering with lead solder, making stained glass, making ammunition and using firing ranges
  - ➤ Leaded gasoline is still used in some race cars, airplanes and off-road vehicles
- **Health Effects**
  - ➤ Linked to cancer in humans
  - ➤ Systems affected:
    - o Neurological: has been shown to reduce IQ in children by minimum of 5 points
    - o Hematological (blood): decreased activity of several heme biosynthesis enzymes at blood levels (PbB) $<10\mu g/dL$
    - o Gastrointestinal: colic in children PbB 60-100$\mu g/dL$
    - o Cardiovascular: elevated blood pressure PbB$<10\mu g/dL$
    - o Kidney: Decreased glomerular filtration rate at mean PbB$<20\mu g/dL$= decreased kidney function

Mercury: Ranked #3 on ATSDR Priority List of Hazardous Substances (2011)

- Mercury, which is everywhere in the environment due to constant off gassing from the earth's crust, exposure is from: 1. Amalgams, 2. Fish, 3. Vaccines [thimerosal preservative is 50% mercury by weight], 4. Pesticides 5. Corn Sweeteners (HFCS-high fructose corn sweeteners)
- According to Health Canada, silver (mercury) amalgams are the largest single source of mercury exposure
- In the FDA's Total Diet Survey, mercury was found in 100% of canned tuna samples (avg. 0.277ppm), frozen cod/haddock fillets (avg. 0.132ppm), canned mushrooms (avg. 0.0298ppm) and shrimp (avg. 0.0281ppm), fish sticks (avg. 0.0254ppm) and crisped rice cereal (avg. 0.0044ppm)
- Nearly all fish contain trace amounts: http://www.mercury-poison.com/fish_list.htm
- Mercury is released into the environment by oil burning, from its use as a fungicide (applied to seeds), from outdoor paint (banned in *indoor* paint in 1990), from processes involving chlorine manufacture and by cremations (a single crematorium estimates the release of more than 5,400 kg of mercury per yr.)
- The U.S. Environment Protection Agency states a maximum ingestion of 5.5 µg/day of mercury for the average American woman of childbearing age. Interestingly, a can of cola has 39 g of HFCS which could contain as much as 22.23 µg of mercury.
- **Health Effects**
  - ➢ Mercury is rapidly absorbed and accumulates in several tissues, leading to increased oxidative damage, mitochondrial dysfunction and cell death
  - ➢ Affects neurological tissue (demyelinates nerve fibers), kidneys and the immune system
  - ➢ Crosses both the Blood Brain Barrier and the placental barrier, present in breast milk
  - ➢ Affects neurotransmitters dopamine, serotonin and norepinephrine
  - ➢ Can remain in the body for decades unless removed
  - ➢ Mercury toxicity can result in:
    - o speech impairment, hearing impairment and sensory disturbances
    - o hand and leg tremors, dizziness, loss of pain sensation, cramping, insomnia
    - o tinnitus, loss of touch sensation, muscular weakness, decreased memory

- ➢ Implicated in Alzheimer's disease and other chronic neurological complaints, possible carcinogen

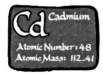

Cadmium: Ranked #7 on ATSDR Priority List of Hazardous Substances (2011)

- • Cadmium is part of the soil and in every form of rock in the environment
- • May be exposed to cadmium in drinking water, food and tobacco
  - ➢ Low levels are found in all foods, highest levels are found in shellfish and organ meats
  - ➢ Found in brilliant paints i.e. cadmium yellow, cadmium red and cadmium orange
- • **Health Effects**
  - ➢ Can severely damage the lungs and is a carcinogen to humans
  - ➢ Eating food or drinking water with very high levels severely irritates the stomach, leading to vomiting and diarrhea
  - ➢ Long-term exposure to lower levels of cadmium in air, food, or water leads to a buildup of cadmium in the kidneys and possibly kidney disease. Other long-term effects can include fragile bones and decreased bone density.

Sources of Heavy Metals:

Heavy metals are a concern for the entire population; we are all exposed to heavy metals daily. In Toronto, the lead pipe replacement program that began in 2010 was later abandoned due to the increased danger of lead in the drinking water. Originally, the city planned to replace the pipe from the street up to the property line, giving homeowners the option to replace the remaining pipe. An environmental engineer provided strong evidence that the joining of the new copper pipes to existing lead pipe, can cause the rusting lead to fall off into the water system.

Water is not the only source of heavy metal contamination. Environmental Defense tested the makeup bags of 6 Canadian women in 2010. The items included foundations, concealers, bronzers, powders, blushes, mascaras, eye liners, eye shadows, lipsticks and glosses. Arsenic was detected in 20%, cadmium in 8% and lead in 96%. Interestingly, the highest levels were found in lip glosses, something that can easily be ingested.

Environmental Defense also conducted research on heavy metals in the Canadian diet. The Total Diet Study and the Metallic Lunch Study indicated alarming amounts of cadmium and lead in food. High levels of mercury can also be found in high fructose corn syrup (HFCS).

Synergistic Effects of Heavy Metals

The synergistic effect of mercury, cadmium and lead is unfortunately just now being investigated and we do know that their effects are more than simply additive. In other words, one plus one does not equal two. One plus one may make 1,000.

Separately, mercury and lead are extremely neurotoxic but combined the negative effects are worsened. An animal study investigated the collective outcome of mercury and lead administration to rodents. A dose of mercury sufficient to kill 1% of tested rats, when combined with a dose of lead sufficient to kill less than 1% of rats, resulted in killing **100%** of the tested rats.

Similar observations are presented in the following chart with aluminum and mercury on nerve cell (neuron) survival. Individually, the neurotoxicity of aluminum revealed a 15% death rate of neurons after 24 hours and mercury a death rate of 70% after 24 hours. When combined, the metals synergistically resulted in a significant death rate of 95% of neurons after 24 hours. Interestingly, aluminum and mercury are used in childhood vaccinations *(please refer to Vaccines for more information)*.

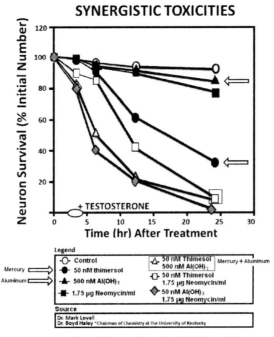

http://homeoint.ru/pdfs/haley.pdf

This suggests that many people are absorbing dangerous levels of metals. The CDC and Health Canada continue to monitor the exposure of the population to environmental chemicals. For more information please refer to: The CDC Fourth National Report on Human Exposure to Environmental Chemicals http://www.cdc.gov/exposurereport/pdf/fourthreport.pdf or The Canadian Health Measures Survey http://www23.statcan.gc.ca/imdb/p2SV.pl?Function= getSurvey&SDDS=5071&Item_Id=129548&lang=en.

The accumulation of heavy metals in the body can have serious health effects. Fortunately, there are treatments, including DMSA, DMPS, EDTA and Therapeutic Fasting that have been used to effectively reduce the burden of heavy metals.

References:
1. http://www.klinghardtacademy.com/Articles/Heavy-Metals-and-Chronic-Diseases.html
2. http://www.hbci.com/~wenonah/hydro/heavmet.htm
3. http://www.cbc.ca/news/technology/story/2011/03/01/tech-mercury-in-depth.html
4. http://www.cbc.ca/news/canada/toronto/story/2010/03/10/lead-pipes.html.
5. http://www.atsdr.cdc.gov/
6. http://environmentaldefence.ca/sites/default/files/report_files/Heavy%20Metals%20Cosmetics%20Factsheet%20FINAL_0.pdf
7. Metallic Lunch: an analysis of Heavy metals in the Canadian diet. Environmental Defense Canada, May 2003. www.edcanada.org
8. Wallinga, D. Institute for Agriculture & Trade Policy. Not So Sweet: Missing Mercury and High Fructose Corn Syrup. 2009.
9. Shubert et al., Combined Effects in Toxicology-A Rapid systematic Testing Procedure: Cadmium, Mercury & Lead. J. of Toxicology & Environmental Health 4:763, 1978.
10. Hayley, B. Mercury toxicity: Genetic susceptibility and synergistic effects. Medical Veritas. 2 (2005) 535–542. http://homeoint.ru/pdfs/haley.pdf

Vaccines

Are you an Informed Consumer?

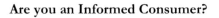

The use of vaccinations for disease prevention began in 1796, when a British physician used diseased matter from a dairymaid infected with cowpox to prevent a healthy young boy from acquiring smallpox. This first example of immunization paved the way for the eradication of many diseases that plagued the population.

Today, the standard Canadian vaccine schedule begins early in your child's life. The types of vaccines have more than doubled since 1980. Today's grandparents received 12 doses of four brands of vaccines while their grandchildren now receive 46-47 doses of fourteen different vaccines in the first 4-6 years of life (8 doses of 3-4 shots are in the first two months). Interestingly, deaths caused by diseases prevented for by vaccines, **declined by 98% prior** to the implementation of this massive schedule. The damage that can occur to the immune system from vaccination is not familiar to many. A healthy immune system has two main parts; TH1, the first response that senses and eliminates organisms causing disease and TH2, which creates the antibodies and the memory of the disease to prevent re-infection. Newborns have an immature immune system in which TH2 dominates. TH1 later takes over as the immune system matures and comes into contact with infectious agents through the nose and mouth. Vaccines however bypass the TH1 mechanism through injection, over stimulating TH2 and confusing the immune system. TH1 can become suppressed resulting in autoimmune disease (e.g. Juvenile diabetes), allergic disorders and frequent infections.

The original concept of immunization was very beneficial in history. Nevertheless, many unforeseen negative impacts have occurred from vaccinations and from their ingredients. In 1959, Bernice Eddy discovered that the Polio vaccine which was intended to protect the population from a contagious intestinal virus that affects the CNS carried an infectious agent capable of causing cancer. The agent was later found to be due to a virus, Simian Virus (SV-40), that infected all the monkeys whose kidneys were used to produce the vaccine. Numerous vaccine ingredients used today continue to be very risky to your health. Preservatives and chemical adjuvants such as aluminum phosphate, phenols (carbolic acid), MSG, formaldehyde, gelatin, etc. are potentially harmful. The flu shot and other vaccines still contain mercury. Exposure to toxins during critical stages of development before two years of age is especially dangerous to the brain. Some vaccines are made using monkey kidney, fetal calf blood, chicken embryos, aborted human fetal lung, yeast, etc. all of which may contain contaminating viruses and proteins. The combinations of the ingredients can bioaccumulate, eventually suppressing the immune system, leading to multiple health issues and developmental disorders.

There remains a definite possibility that previously rare conditions could be contributed to by vaccinations. Adverse health events may not be reported or recognized especially when the occurrence is months to years following a vaccination. According to the Public Health Agency of Canada (PHAC), a limited range of adverse events are acceptable only if they occur shortly after the injection.

Studies to compare the long-term health of vaccinated versus unvaccinated people have never been done, nor have studies demonstrating benefit from the cumulative effects of so many vaccines been completed. Vaccinations are **NOT** mandatory in Canada. Three provinces require proof of immunization for school entrance. In Ontario diphtheria, tetanus, polio, measles, mumps and rubella are the immunizations asked for but exceptions are permitted on medical or religious grounds or for reasons of conscience. It is not compulsory legislation.

If your child suffers a negative side effect from a vaccine it is very difficult to place blame on the company that produced the injection; they are very well protected by the government. **In February 2011, the US Supreme Court ruled that the Federal Statute protects vaccine manufacturers from most lawsuits filed by parents who claim their child was harmed. The 1986 National Childhood Vaccine Injury Act, minimized manufacturers from any liability for an adverse reaction suffered following vaccination.** The passage of this act caused a proliferation of new vaccines due to near zero liability and maximum profitability. **The act "leaves a regulatory vacuum in which no one ensures that vaccine manufacturers adequately take account of scientific and technological advancements when designing or distributing their products" (Justice Sonia Sotomayor and joined by Justice Ruth Bader Ginsbur).** This act demonstrates that vaccine manufacturers have near zero accountability because of limited liability. This is very alarming considering we have a tendency to trust that our medications should be helping us and not harming us. Of course, we would like to know that the medication is effective, safe and well researched and not just thrown together to make a profit since minimal liability of the manufacture exists. The act is worded in a manner, that as long as the manufacturers demonstrate that their design is sound and the reaction could not be avoided, they are not liable. You are not prevented from entering into a lawsuit; however it does make the process for achieving success difficult and convoluted.

There is a fair amount of controversy that exists around vaccinations. The opinions of whether double the amounts of immunizations are a necessity are questionable. Dr. Paul Offit, USA's foremost advocate of vaccines claims that children are so resilient that you should not worry about vaccinations. He further believes that infants "theoretically have the capacity to respond to about 10,000 vaccines at once". Considering the many documented adverse reactions and the knowledge about the immature immune system of a newborn, one can question what is Dr. Offit basing his conclusions on? At NaturoMedic.com we follow the precautionary principle, an ethical guideline that helps us select whether or not a treatment should be done when the risks are not known. In regards to vaccines, we recommend extreme caution when vaccinating your children with potentially harmful substances before their immune system has had the opportunity to develop.

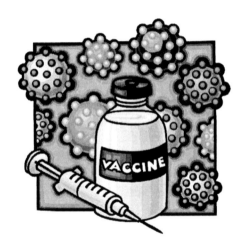

Vaccine Ingredient	Information/Adverse Effect	Vaccine	Interesting Fact
Thimerosal (Mercury)	•Previously widely used but later removed from some products •Causes neurological disabilities in children •2007 PHAC states little is known about the ethylmercury from thimerosal, whether similar to neurotoxin or crosses blood brain barrier but presumed to be excreted by bowels •**Contains 50% Mercury by weight and 50% formaldehyde (a neurotoxin).**	•Influenza vaccines Fluviral® and Vaxigrip® •Tetanus Toxoid •Recombivax HB® (hepatitis B) •Menomune® A/C/Y/W-135 (meningococcal vaccine) •Trace amounts in: Infanrix™-hexa (6 given to newborns), Engerix®-B (hepatitis B) and Twinrix® (hepatitis A & B)	•**Pregnant women advised against consuming fish with mercury and cautioned about dental fillings (silver mercury amalgams) to protect unborn infant but encouraged to receive mercury filled flu shot** More Info: •PHAC - July 1, 2007 - Thimerosal updated statement. http://www.phac-aspc.gc.ca/publicat/ccdr-rmtc/07vol33/acs-06/index-eng.php •Film produced by University of Calgary showing how mercury causes brain neuron degeneration. http://movies.commons.ucalgary.ca/mercury/
Aluminum	•Commonly used •Used to provoke a sustained immune response •**Neurotoxin**	•DPT (diphtheria, pertussis, tetanus) •Hepatitis A and B •Pneumococcal vaccines •Meningococcal vaccines	http://www.iaomt.org/testfoundation/aluminumvaccines.htm

Ingredient	Information/Adverse Effect	Vaccine	Interesting Fact
Biological ingredients	•Certain lab-altered viruses and bacteria toxins or parts of viruses and bacteria are used to produce immunity •Human fetal tissue which has replaced contaminated monkey tissue may induce DNA mutations contributing to children's autism •**2011, HPV vaccine found to be contaminated with recombinant HPV DNA (actual virus) from its genetically engineered "virus-like particles'**	•Live virus vaccines: MMR, & chickenpox •Chicken Embryos: Influenza and MMRII •Fetal calf tissue: Chicken pox & Pediacel® (diphtheria, tetanus, pertussis, polio and Hib)	•Health Canada has found it necessary to test vaccines made from bovine (cow tissue) for mad cow disease but not every single dose is tested •In 2010 two pig viruses contaminated the rotavirus vaccine (Rota Teq); one causes immune suppression and death in baby pigs but was still approved for use in humans in Canada and added to vaccine schedule in 2011.

Vaccine	Information	Adverse Reaction
MMR: Measles, Mumps, Rubella		
Measles	• **Does not confer permanent immunity. In large outbreaks over 95% of cases have a history of vaccination** • **World Health Organization-15x more likely to contract measles by being vaccinated against the disease than by those who aren't vaccinated**	• Encephalitis • Subacute sclerosing panencephalitis • Guillain-Barre syndrome • Febrile and afebrile convulsions • Seizures, ataxia, ocular palsies, anaphylaxis, edema, bronchial spasm
Mumps	• Contagious virus beginning with a fever, headache, muscle aches and fatigue • Symptoms usually disappear within a week • When contracted in prepubescent childhood it is rarely harmful and provides lifelong immunity • When contracted as an adult can typically cause one teste or one ovary to become sterile in 30% of cases	• 1993, prestigious Medical Journal, the Lancet published data confirming aseptic meningitis as a recognized complication of mumps vaccine, **15 to 35** days after the shot
Rubella	• German measles, contagious virus causing slight fever, rash, sore throat and runny nose. Lymph nodes on the back of the head, behind the ears and on the side of the neck may become tender • Treatment consists of allowing the disease to run its course • Medical intervention is seldom required, symptoms usually disappear within a few days • **The infection has adverse effects for Pregnant women and their unborn child.** • 1979, Wistar RA27/3 strain vaccine produced from cell lines obtained from the tissue of aborted fetuses	• 1993 Japan removes MMR vaccine from the market because it was causing encephalitis in 1 of every 1044 people vaccinated • Drug company has an extensive list of ailments known to occur following the MMR shot

Vaccine	Information	Adverse Reaction
Varicella	• Chicken pox vaccine • **"Vaccine not recommend as infection with chicken pox early in life will help to develop antibodies to help fight infections at a later stage"** Dr. Sadbhavna Pandit, Senior Medical Officer Paediatrics, Groves Memorial Community Hospital	• Vaccine Adverse Event Reporting System received 67.5 adverse event reports per 100,000 doses of chicken pox vaccine sold between March 1995 and July 1998 • **4 percent of cases (about 1 in 33,000 doses) were serious, including shock, convulsions, encephalitis, thrombocytopenia and 14 deaths.** • 17 adverse events now added to the manufacturer's product label since 1995: secondary bacterial infections (cellulitis), secondary transmission (infection of close contacts), transverse myelitis, Guillain Barre Syndrome and herpes zoster (shingles).
Priorix-Tetra: Measles Mumps Rubella Varicella	• Approved 2010 to replace 2 shots of MMR and varicella (chickenpox) • Measles and mumps are cultured in chick embryo cells • Rubella and varicella are cultured on cells derived from lung tissue of an aborted human baby	• Live virus capable of causing infections: "rash, including measles-like, rubella-like and varicella-like rash" occur in 1-10% of 9-27 month old children after vaccination • Transmission of varicella virus may occur to others after developing a rash following the vaccination • Throat excretion of the rubella virus is known to occur about 7 to 28 days after vaccination • Bleeding or bruising more easily, Kawasaki syndrome (fever, rash on the trunk, peeling of skin on hands and fingers, swollen glands in the neck, red eyes, lips, throat and tongue), meningitis, arthralgia and arthritis, encephalitis, Guillain Barré syndrome, peripheral neuritis, anaphylaxis.

Vaccine	Information	Adverse Reaction
Gardasil	• Prevention of infection caused by Human Papilloma Virus (HPV) types 6, 11, 16, and 18 (capable of causing cancer) in young girls ages 9-26 • No testing has been done on ages 9-12 years • **Maximum follow up study is four years however, the time course from CIN III (cervical dysplasia) to invasive cancer averages between 8.1 to 12.6 years therefore questionable whether can prevent cervical cancer.** • Cervical cancer was once a leading cause of cancer death for women, however in the past forty years, both the incidence and the number of deaths from it have decreased, largely because of Pap screening • 2010 Health Canada approved use of Gardasil® for boys and men aged 9-26 years • 2011 US FDA rejected Merck's fourth application to extend its Gardasil™ licence to use in US women ages 27-45 but was approved by Canada	• **2008 FDA Statement on Gardasil™: 73.3% of girls in the clinical trials developed "new medical conditions" post vaccination and 17 girls died** • Pre-licensure clinical trials were only tested in fewer than 100 girls 16 years and younger; reports of 9 deaths, 3 blood clots, 4 cardiac arrests, 9 cases of lupus, 6 strokes, and 2 cases of vasculitis • Thirteen vials of the Gardasil HPV4 vaccine currently on the market worldwide have been found contaminated with recombinant HPV DNA • Dr. Sin Hang Lee (a pathologist) analyzed samples after young girl developed HPV and acute onset Juvenile Rheumatoid Arthritis, within 24 hours of her third injection. Recombinant HPV DNA was later found in the girl's blood two years after that injection; this is significant because natural HPV is normally on the skin and membranes and does not survive in the bloodstream • Thousands of reports of problems from facial nerve paralysis to pancreatitis, exacerbation of HPV symptoms -- outbreaks of warts and precancerous lesions. And now, 26 deaths are associated with the vaccine

Vaccine	Information	Adverse Reaction
Haemophilus Influenza B (Hib)	• A bacteria that can cause upper respiratory and ear infections, pneumonia, epiglottis, septic arthritis and meningitis.	• **In 1996-2001, ⅔ of H. influenzae invasive disease was caused by non-b serotypes and leading to significant morbidity and mortality. There are no vaccines for the non-b serotypes of H.influenzae disease.** *'Invasive Infections Caused by Haemophilus influenzae Serotypes in Twelve Canadian IMPACT Centers, 1996-2001'* • adverse reactions reported include: Guillain-Barre syndrome (an autoimmune illness characterized by paralysis and demyelination of the nerve sheaths), transverse myelitis (paralyzing disease of the spinal cord), and thrombocytopenia (a blood disorder causing clotting and spontaneous bleeding, usually internally-bruising).
Pediacel®: **Diphtheria** **Tetanus** **Pertussis** **Polio** **Hib**	• In Canadian childhood vaccination programs, vaccines against diphtheria, tetanus, pertussis (whooping cough), polio and Haemophilus (a bacterial infection) are administered as one shot • Diptheria is a contagious bacterial disease of respiratory system treatable with common antibiotic • Pertussis is a respiratory disease, rarely fatal but considered life threatening to infants under 6 months • Polio is an intestinal virus that may attack nerve cells of the brain and spinal cord. • Tetanus is non-contagious disease that causes severe muscular contractions and lock jaw	• 1975 FDA concluded diphtheria vaccine is not as effective as anticipated and may still occur in vaccinated individuals • Pertussis and diphtheria deaths were rapidly declining well before the use of DTP in the late 1940s. Despite its use for more than six decades in one form or another, whooping cough outbreaks still occur in highly vaccinated populations. • **In 1985, Centre for Disease Control reported that 87% of polio in the U.S. was caused by the vaccine** • In Canada, 5 cases of tetanus occur annually with no deaths recorded since 1991. Severe fatal neurological and paralytic disorders have been linked to tetanus vaccine.

Vaccine	Information	Adverse Reaction
H1N1 (Swine Flu)	• Swine flu, a subtype of Influenza A virus • **2000-8000 Canadians die each year due to influenza and about 250 000 to 500 000 die each year from seasonal flu worldwide.** • **Nov. 5 2009, During the "global pandemic" there have been a total of 115 deaths in Canada due to H1N1 and 4,000 around the world** • In Mexico 2009 there were 11 attributable deaths when the panic broke out over this new flu infection	• All flu vaccines contain thimerosol (mercury) and formaldehyde • No clinical data on children ages 10-17 years and elderly over 60 years • may not fully protect all people who are vaccinated • **WHO changed the definition of pandemic and lowered the threshold for declaration allowing for the transformation of relatively mild flu into a worldwide pandemic, to implement relevant plans and the use of pandemic vaccines.** • Have a higher risk than usual flu vaccines, as adjuvants that are known to stimulate the immune system are used and can cause autoimmune disease and immunological complications. New procedures were allowed using fast growing cancer like cells. The potential for these proteins when injected to cause cancer has never been excluded by clinical testing.

61

References:

1. Miller N. Vaccines are they really safe? New Atlantean Press, Santa Fe, New Mexico. 2009
2. Immunization in Canada; May, 1997; Vol 23S4
3. http://www.phac-aspc.gc.ca/publicat/cig-gci/p01-tab01-eng.php
4. http://www.gsk.ca/english/docs-pdf/Priorix_tetra_2010.pdf
5. http://vran.org/in-the-news/potential-bio-hazard-found-in-gardasil-vaccine/
6. http://vran.org/about-vaccines/specific-vaccines/polio-vaccine/sv-40-contamination-of-polio-virus-vaccines/
7. http://www.expressindia.com/latest-news/Vaccines-weather-to-blame-for-rising-chicken-pox-cases/334700/
8. www.nvic.org
9. http://vran.org/about-vaccines/specific-vaccines/diphtheria-tetanus-pertussis-hib-vaccine/
10. http://vran.org/about-vaccines/specific-vaccines/diphtheria-tetanus-pertussis-hib-vaccine/haemophilus-influenza-b-hib-the-disease-the-vaccine/
11. http://www.vaccineinfo.net/immunization/vaccine/hpv/doc_against_HPV.shtml
12. http://boards.medscape.com/forums?128@884.nuVcaMCbCbz@.29efea0e!comment=1
13. Hikel, K. High Court Protects Vaccine Makers for 'Unavoidable' Adverse Events. http://www.medscape.com/viewarticle/737900
14. http://vran.org/about-vaccines/specific-vaccines/

Microorganisms

Do we live with or without them?

A microorganism is a tiny life form that cannot be seen by the human eye. These organisms are found everywhere on Earth. They are present in the air, water, soil, plants, animals and even in and on the human body. In fact, microbial cells on our bodies are estimated to outnumber human cells ten to one. Now this does not mean that we are full of germs and need to purify ourselves. There are many beneficial bacteria that the body needs to function properly and to help protect us. For instance, in our digestive system we have trillions of beneficial flora (bacteria) from mouth to rectum. These bacteria produce enzymes that help break down proteins, carbohydrates, fiber and fats. They create substances that assist the transport of vitamins and minerals through the gut for absorption in our blood stream. They can also synthesize essential nutrients including vitamin B1, B2, B3, B5, B6, B12, folic acid, vitamin K2 and some amino acids. These beneficial bacteria are important for maintaining good health and a strong immune system. Below is a small list of beneficial microbes found in the body.

MICROBES IN THE HEALTHY HUMAN BODY*	
Microbe found in:	
Ear (outer)	*Aspergillus* (fungus)
Skin	*Candida* (fungus)
Small intestine	*Clostridium*
Intestines	*Escherichia coli*
Vagina	*Gardnerella vaginalis*
Stomach	*Lactobacillus*
Urethra	*Mycobacterium*
Nose	*Staphylococcus aureus*
Eye	*Staphylococcus epidermis*
Mouth	*Streptococcus salivarius*
Large intestine	*Trichomonas hominis* (protozoa)

*A selection of usually harmless microbes, some of which help keep our bodies functioning normally. If their numbers become unbalanced, however, these microbes may make us sick. All are bacteria, unless otherwise noted.

http://biomicrobials.com/health.html

It is important to maintain a good balance of beneficial bacteria, not only in the digestive system but throughout the whole body. Overgrowth of these bacteria or invasion of other microorganisms can lead to disease. Microorganisms could be a bacteria, parasite, virus, mould or fungus that the immune system recognizes as a foreign substance.

In the body when a foreign substance invades (also known as an antigen), several immune cells work together to recognize and respond. Antibodies, which are designed to identify and neutralize the problem, are triggered by specialized white blood cells (lymphocytes) to lock onto the antigen. Once activated, the antibodies continue to exist in the body so that if the same antigen invades again, the antibody is ready to do their job and prevent you from getting sick. This is also the principle that immunizations are based on. The eradication of smallpox was the first example of an immunization. An English physician, Edward Jenner, in 1796 observed that milkmaids who developed cowpox did not develop the deadly small pox. When the milkmaids were exposed to the cowpox virus their immune systems created antibodies to the antigen on the cowpox virus. These antigens being similar to the smallpox virus allowed the immune system to recognize and neutralize small pox as they both are from the same viral family *(please refer to Vaccines for more information)*.

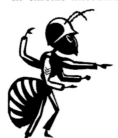

In chronic infections, microorganisms have the ability to evade the immune system; they can hide in areas of poor circulation, create an environment that promotes their growth and dominate the host's behavior. The ability of microorganisms to control the host's body can be seen in "zombie ants". A newfound fungus, *Ophiocordyceps camponoti-balzani*, has the ability to infect an ant, take over its brain and then kill the ant once it moves to an area that is ideal for the fungi to grow and spread its spores to other ants. The fungus actually sticks out of the ants head and controls their body movements. This mind control fungus has not been found to affect humans but microorganisms are capable of affecting our mind and body. Neuropeptides released by microorganisms can influence behavior i.e. increase cravings for sugar consumption to support the microbes. Research has implicated specific infections as risk factors in the occurrence of schizophrenia. These include rubella, influenza, chicken pox, *herpes* (HSV-2), polio, *coxsackie* virus, Lyme disease and Toxoplasmosis. The association of schizophrenia with these microbes suggests that these organisms have stealth capabilities and are not fully eliminated by the immune system.

Stealth microorganisms should not be confused with antimicrobial resistant microorganisms. Resistant microbes are able to withstand treatment from antimicrobial medicines. Standard treatments become ineffective and the infection persists. For example, MRSA (Methicillin-resistant *Staphylococcous aureus*) is a highly resistant bacterium to the traditional treatment of methicillin and therefore persists in the body. This form of resistance is believed to be the result of the misuse of antimicrobial medicines whereby the organism mutates to become a superbug and is no longer threatened by the same drug treatment. Stealth microorganisms are different in that they have the ability to survive in the body even after our immune system mounts an attack against it.

These stealth microorganisms are very difficult to detect by Western Science and can often be mislabeled as an autoimmune disease. The body attacks itself, attempting to remove the stealth organism. Unfortunately, healthy tissues are often affected, weakening the body. In Multiple Sclerosis, *herpes virus 6, mycoplasmas, borrelia, cytomegalovirus* and Lyme have been identified as suspected causes. Stealth microorganisms have also been acknowledged in osteoarthritis, Parkinson's disease, Lou Gehrig's disease and cancer. With a weakened immune system, these microorganisms can persist and lead to disease.

There are multiple body and lifestyle factors that can contribute to the weakening of the immune system, disturbing the balance of beneficial flora, creating an environment for foreign substances to invade and grow. For example, gut bacteria grow well at normal body temperature (37°C), but bacteria from plants may be killed at that temperature. Therefore someone who has a low temperature may have an increased risk for opportunistic infection of stealth microorganisms. In 2008 the Human Microbiome Project (HMP) was launched. This five year project was initiated to characterize and analyze the role of human microbes in health and disease. The results can help not only with methods to optimize health but they also can potentially help with identifying predisposition and susceptibility to disease. It is important to be aware of both the good and the harmful microorganisms in our environment that have an influence on our overall health.

References:
1.   http://www.purenewyou.com/shop/index.php?main_page=index&cPath=162
2.   http://www.safewater.org/PDFS/resourcesknowthefacts/Disease_Causing_Micro Org.pdf
3.   World Health Organization: www.who.int
4.   http://commonfund.nih.gov/hmp/overview.aspx
5.   http://news.nationalgeographic.com/news/2011/03/pictures/110303-zombie-ants-fungus-new-species-fungi-bugs-science-brazil/
6.   http://www.dailymail.co.uk/sciencetech/article-1386717/Why-zombie-ants-infected-mind-controlling-fungus-kill-high-noon.html
7.   http://www.ncbi.nlm.nih.gov/pmc/articles/PMC3335463/

Weather

A front is coming

It is well documented that changes in temperature and weather can have an effect on physiological processes in the body. We have all experienced an increase in perspiration when there is too much heat or shivering when we are too cold. Throughout history the weather has been connected to many health related ailments.

In 400 BC, the Greek physician Hippocrates taught about the direct effects of humidity and weather on certain medical conditions including migraines, arthritis and respiratory difficulties. Today, approximately 12% of the population suffers from migraine headaches and over 50% of these migraines are triggered by sensitivity to weather changes.

There are many ways in which the weather can affect physiological processes in the body. For example, when we are hot, sweat evaporates from your skin to help cool you down and when we are cold, shivering causes muscle twitches that help generate heat for the body. In extreme heat conditions, the heart rate rises and blood vessels dilate to allow more blood to reach the skin's surface (blushing). On the other hand, in extreme cold our bodies constrict blood vessels to keep heat inside. These basic principles can help explain how migraines and arthritic pain can be affected by changes in the weather.

As pressure and temperature rises, blood vessels in the head can either contract or dilate to compensate for alterations in oxygen levels. Expanded blood vessels increase pressure on nerve fibers, triggering migraine pain. Barometric receptors in the brain can also increase vasodilation of blood vessels in the head with pressure changes. In the brain, there are numerous cavities and chambers filled with fluid or air. Pressure differences between trapped air in the sinuses and the air outside can also lead to pain when the nasal cavities are blocked. For example, if the barometric pressure drops, a headache or migraine can be triggered in a person who has a stuffy nose.

Many researchers believe that it is a variety of weather factors and not pressure alone that triggers weather related headaches. For example, bright sunlight, high humidity, dry air and windy or stormy weather can all play a role. The degree of sensitivity can vary with each person, although the most important factor is **change** in weather, regardless of fluctuations in humidity, temperature or pressure.

Research overwhelmingly supports the sensitivity to weather amongst people with arthritis. An increase in pain is more often reported on cold, damp days that have rapidly falling barometric pressure. Some people, depending on the type of arthritic pain, can sense in advance the upcoming weather. In 1961, J. Hollander M.D., a specialist in arthritis, demonstrated that high humidity combined with low barometric pressure led to an increase in joint pain and stiffness. He theorized that inflamed joints swell as pressure drops, which irritates the nerves around joints and puts pressure on the tissue. Additional theories exist on the mechanisms that result in pain in the body due to weather changes. One theory explains how bones and muscles have different densities and during alterations in temperature or humidity, the inflamed/injured joint and muscle will unequally expand or contract and increase pain.

Cold and dampness appear to be the main factors in the Great Lakes region. From a Traditional Chinese Medicine (TCM) perspective, these are two environmental factors that play a part in disease. Cold and Dampness are known n TCM as two of 5 Pernicious External Disease Factors (Dry, Heat & Wind are also included). Cold invasion in the body can lead to severe sharp pain, while Dampness causes swelling, heaviness, stiffness and soreness of the joints. These two climatic phenomena are known to externally influence arthritic pain. Interestingly, an "Aches and Pain" forecast for your area can be found by logging onto the Weather Channel's website (http://www.weather.com/activities/health/achesandpains/).

Considerable research has shown that asthmatic conditions can be affected by many weather situations. Extreme hot or cold temperatures, changes in barometric pressure, humidity, wind, dry and damp air have all been found to affect respiratory function and increase asthmatic symptoms.

It is clear that the daily changes to the weather can influence our overall function and health. Are you affected by the weather? Does cold bother you? Do you get brain freeze easily? Does shopping in the frozen food section in summer bother you? Do you hate the cold? Do you always have cold fingers and toes? Do your symptoms get worse with air conditioning? Does your arthritis get worse on cold damp days? Do your joints swell in damp weather? Does the change in temperature give you headaches or migraines? Do you get tired with weather changes? These are just a few symptoms that are caused by sensitivities to weather and temperature. Treatments for cold, heat, wind, dampness and humidity are all available at NaturoMedic.com to remove the disease factor.

References:

1. http://www.bbc.co.uk/weather/weatherwise/living/effects/
2. http://www.relieve-migraine-headache.com/barometric-pressure-headache.html
3. http://www.mayoclinic.com/health/headaches/AN00751
4. http://www.asthmainformationguide.com/asthma-and-weather
5. http://www.barometricpressureheadache.com/forecasting-the-weather/
6. http://www.manfredkaiser.com/rheumatism.html
7. Kaptchuk, T. The Web That Has No Weaver. Methuen Publications, Agincourt, Ontario. 1983.

Radiation and Electromagnetic Fields

What is your Dose?

What is radiation?

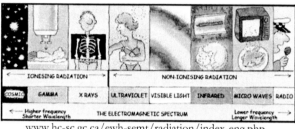

www.hc-sc.gc.ca/ewh-semt/radiation/index-eng.php

Radiation is often described as energetic particles or waves travelling through a substance or space. There are many different kinds of radiation, both natural and manmade in origin. There are two broad categories of radiation: ionizing and non-ionizing. When people talk about radiation they are usually referring to ionizing radiation, radiation strong enough to knock an electron off of an atom. Examples of this can be found in nature including cosmic radiation from outer space or radioactive materials naturally occurring in the earth. These forms of radiation make up what is known as background radiation. Humans not only get exposed to this type of radiation, we also contribute to ionizing radiation (higher frequency and shorter wavelength) when running common medical diagnostics like x-rays. Non-ionizing radiation on the other hand, does not carry enough energy to completely remove an electron from an atom. There are many examples of non-ionizing radiation (lower frequency and longer wavelength) in our environment, including ultraviolet radiation from the sun, light, heat, microwaves and radio waves.

How is radiation harmful?

Non-ionizing radiation does have its dangers with over exposure. For example spending too much time in the sun will cause our skin to burn.

Discussions around the dangers of radiation exposure often refer to ionizing radiation. This type of radiation causes physical damage to living tissue. When electrons are "knocked" from atoms, the atom becomes excited and attempts to interact with another atom. These interactions can produce free radicals that damage important molecules and cellular DNA, eventually leading to tissue destruction. DNA is the blueprint to make new cells. If it is damaged, the newly produced cells may not function properly and tumor growth can occur. Large doses of exposure at one time, like after nuclear accidents or fallout from weapons, can cause radiation sickness, cataracts, hair loss, sterility, burns, loss of thyroid function and death. Children are more susceptible to radiation because

69

they are growing rapidly, more cell divisions are taking place and there is a higher chance for damage to occur. That is also why x-rays are not performed on women who are pregnant.

Radiation in Medicine

Radiation is used in medicine for many tests, the most common being x-rays, cat-scans, mammograms and nuclear medicine (where radioactive material is injected into the body). The degree of radiation exposure with each test varies greatly. There is no conclusive evidence that having a single radiological test will cause problems, but having repeated tests does increase people's exposure to above normal levels of background radiation. The benefit of a proper diagnosis has to be weighed against the risk of the radiation exposure.

Typical Effective Radiation Dose from Diagnostic X Ray—Single Exposure

Exam	Effective Dose mSv (mrem)[1]	Exam	Effective Dose mSv (mrem)[2]
Chest (LAT)	0.04 (4)	Mammogram (four views)	0.7 (70)
Chest (AP)	0.02 (2)	Dental (lateral)	0.02 (2)
Skull (AP)	0.03 (3)	Dental (panoramic)	0.09 (9)
Skull (Lat)	0.01 (1)	DEXA (whole body)	0.0004 (0.04)
Pelvis (AP)	0.7 (70)	Hip	0.8 (80)
Thoracic Spine (AP)	0.4 (40)	Hand or Foot	0.005 (0.5)
Lumbar Spine (AP)	0.7 (70)	Abdomen	1.2 (120)

http://hps.org/documents/meddiagimaging.pdf

Complete Exams	Effective Dose mSv (mrem)[1]
Intravenous Pyelogram (kidneys, 6 films)	2.5 (250)
Barium Swallow (24 images, 106 sec. fluoroscopy)	1.5 (150)
Barium Enema (10 images, 137 sec. fluoroscopy)	7.0 (700)
CT Head	2.0 (200)
CT Chest	8.0 (800)
CT Abdomen	10.0 (1,000)
CT Pelvis	10.0 (1,000)
Angioplasty (heart study)	7.5 (750) - 57.0 (5,700)[3]
Coronary Angiogram	4.6 (460) - 15.8 (1,580)[3]

http://hps.org/documents/meddiagimaging.pdf

Nuclear Medicine Scan	Radiopharmaceutical (common trade name)	Effective Dose mSv (mrem)[2]
Brain (PET)	^{15}O water	1.0 (100)
Brain (perfusion)	^{99m}Tc HMPAO	6.9 (690)
Hepatobiliary (liver flow)	^{99m}Tc Sulfur Colloid	2.8 (280)
Bone	^{99m}Tc MDP	4.2 (420)
Lung Perfusion/Ventilation	^{99m}Tc MAA & ^{133}Xe	2.0 (200)
Kidney (filtration rate)	^{99m}Tc DTPA	3.6 (360)
Kidney (tubular function)	^{99m}Tc MAG3	5.2 (520)
Tumor/Infection	^{67}Ga	18.5 (1,850)
Heart (rest)	^{99m}Tc sestimibi (Cardiolite)	6.7 (670)
Heart (stress)	^{99m}Tc sestimibi (Cardiolite)	5.85 (585)
Heart	^{201}Tl chloride	11.8 (1,180)
Heart (rest)	^{99m}Tc tetrofosmin (Myoview)	5.6 (560)
Heart (stress)	^{99m}Tc tetrofosmin (Myoview)	5.6 (560)
Various PET Studies	^{18}F FDG	14.0 (1,400)

http://hps.org/documents/meddiagimaging.pdf

In conclusion, radiation is all around us. Both ionizing and non-ionizing radiation can cause damage if over-exposed. The most dangerous exposure would be from acute high dose exposure after a major accident such as a nuclear reactor melt down. The most serious problem with long-term exposure to low doses of radiation is the development of cancer.

Check out this **free** app from iTunes to calculate your exposure: **My Radiation**

Electromagnetic Fields

Electromagnetic fields (EMFs) represent a growing environmental influence. All populations are exposed to varying amounts of EMFs. According to the World Health Organization (WHO) the levels will continue to increase with advances in technology. Some current sources include video display units (VDUs) associated with computers, mobile phones and their base stations. The exposure to EMFs is growing exponentially, creating different perspectives and controversy on the health implications.

The health effects of mobile phones are an increasing concern. Numerous studies have investigated the effects of radiofrequency fields on brain electrical activity, cognitive function and sleep. Tissue heating is the principal short-term interaction between radiofrequencies and the human body. To date, research does not suggest consistent evidence of adverse effects although concerns have been raised. Most energy is absorbed by the skin and other superficial tissues; the resulting temperature rise in the brain or organs is understood to be negligible.

71

Long-term research has mainly focused on potential risks with brain tumours. There are some indications of increased risk associated with cumulative hours of cell phone use (reported in a retrospective case-control study on adults, INTERPHONE, coordinated by the International Agency for Research on Cancer). Researchers concluded that biases and errors limit the strength of the study, therefore preventing a causal relationship. The WHO does mention that these many limitations **cannot completely rule out negative health implications from cellular phones**.

Electromagnetic hypersensitivity is a variety of non-specific symptoms reported by individuals following exposure to EMFs. Dermatological symptoms, including redness, tingling and burning sensations, are the most commonly reported. In addition fatigue, tiredness, dizziness, nausea and heart palpitations have been experienced. Currently, the collection of these symptoms are not a recognized syndrome, much like fibromyalgia, chronic fatigue syndrome and multiple chemical sensitivities were not recognized.

While the increased risk of brain tumours with the rising use of mobile phones is lacking in the data, further research is necessary. The WHO has also recommended exploring the health effects of longer life time exposure (over 15 years) to children and adolescents.

At NaturoMedic.com, we believe that the cumulative exposure to these fields, not merely cell phones, does play a contributory role to disease, especially when other disease causing factors are present. For example, the presence of mercury fillings in conjunction with EMFs can create a cumulative significant health challenge.

References:
1. www.hc-sc.gc.ca/ewh-semt/radiation/index-eng.php
2. www.health.ny.gov/publications/4402/
3. epa.gov/radiation/understand/health_effects.html
4. **My Radiation**: Free application from iTunes
5. World Health Organization: http://www.who.int/peh-emf/en/
6. http://www.who.int/mediacentre/factsheets/fs193/en/index.html

Chapter 4

Disease Causing Factors: Lifestyle

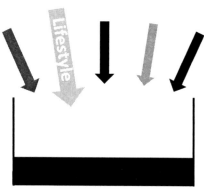

Challenging Habits

Alcohol

Cheers and Tears

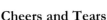

There are numerous studies suggesting moderate alcohol consumption can have protective benefits against heart disease by raising HDL (good) cholesterol and reducing plaque accumulation in the arteries. Currently, an official safe amount of alcohol does not exist yet most studies suggest one drink or less daily. Unfortunately, the average person consuming alcohol does not stop at one drink per day.

A drink is considered to be 12 oz. of beer or 5 oz. of wine or 1.5 oz. of 80-proof distilled spirits. Drinking more than 3 drinks per day or drinking heavily at one time has direct toxic effects on the body.

Ethanol (alcohol) is metabolized by the liver and converted to an aldehyde product that is believed to be responsible for the harmful effects to the body. The process results in the production of free radicals that can further damage the heart, the liver and many other systems. This can lead to hypertension, cardiomyopathy, congestive heart failure, stroke, fatty infiltration of the liver, inflammation, cirrhosis and immunosuppression. In addition, food cravings often occur while consuming alcohol, as the body enters a state of reactive hypoglycemia. The drop in blood sugar can lead to anxiety, dizziness, depression, visual disturbances and heart palpitations. A number of cancers of the mouth, throat, stomach, colon and breast have been linked to increased alcohol consumption.

Intake of alcohol can impair digestion and cause malabsorption of important nutrients. Alcohol is absorbed through the stomach and intestines into the bloodstream. Ethanol can damage the lining of the stomach, prevent the secretion of digestive enzymes from the pancreas and impair transport of the nutrients. Many nutritional deficiencies, especially vitamin B1, can result, leading to very serious health consequences.

Dehydration often occurs with alcohol consumption as alcohol is a diuretic, causing the increase of fluid loss from the body and potassium excretion. Thirst, muscle cramps, dizziness and faintness can result with alterations in potassium balance and water loss. Also, alterations in fluid and acid-base balance from alcohol consumption are important to monitor as increases in acid accumulate in the stomach with alcohol consumption contributes to changes in the acid-base balance. The pH of the body which refers to the homeostasis of all the fluids should remain alkaline (7.37 and 7.43). When the pH falls below 7, decreased organ function, respiratory depression and even death may result.

It is well known that alcohol can be addictive and it is often perceived to be a stimulant. Interestingly, it is actually classified as a general anesthetic and produces a depressive and desensitizing effect on the central nervous system. With continuous consumption, tolerance develops as the brain adapts to diminish the effect, while the liver increases its capability to metabolize alcohol more quickly. These changes in the body create what are known as high functioning alcoholics. Although large quantities of alcohol have been consumed motor control and cognitive function appear to be maintained while in this state. This level of functioning is not preserved during periods of withdrawal.

Alcohol is a psychoactive drug that affects both individual and social development. According to the World Health Organization, it results in 2.5 million deaths globally per year. It affects your senses, thoughts, emotions, behavior and it causes harm to the well-being and health of the people around you. An intoxicated person is at increased risk for violent behavior and risk of injury or death from a motor vehicle accident. MADD (Mothers Against Drunk Driving) Canada estimates that there are 1,350-1,600 impaired crash fatalities in Canada each year (3.7-4.4 deaths per day) from motor vehicle and boating accidents and approximately 73,120 injuries from impaired driving crashes (roughly 200 per day). The harmful impact of alcohol is more than an individual concern; it affects society as a whole.

Many people associate their alcohol consumption with social activities and rarely does this consist of a single drink. As of May 1, 2009 in Ontario, if you are caught driving with a blood alcohol concentration (BAC) from 0.05 to 0.08, the police can immediately suspend your license for 3-30 days.

At NaturoMedic.com, we are not against the consumption of alcohol but for its use in moderation. If you are going to drink: Drink Responsibly!

References:
1. www.who.org
2. http://forcon.ca/learning/alcohol.html
3. http://alcoholism.about.com/cs/alerts/l/blnaa35.htm
4. http://www.mto.gov.on.ca/english/safety/impaired/fact-sheet.shtml
5. http://madd.ca/english/research/magnitudememo.html

Coffee

Caffeine Mon Amore

Coffee is one of the most popular beverages in the world. It is widely known for its energizing effects from a substance known as caffeine. It is not the most harmful beverage to consume and in fact has many health benefits, but as with most things moderation is key. Coffee aggravates certain conditions such as stomach ulcers, heartburn, gallstones, arrhythmias and can cause sleep disturbances or migraines.

Benefits:

1. Source of antioxidants to help prevent cell damage.
2. Reduces risk of certain diseases: Type 2 diabetes, Parkinson's, Alzheimer's, liver cirrhosis.
3. Coffee has been used to help treat spasmodic asthma.
4. Caffeine and methylxanthine, both found in coffee, are metabolic stimulants, which could be helpful in weight loss.
5. Previously used in enemas to enhance peristalsis (movement in the colon) and cause the release of bile containing fat-soluble toxins.

Problems Associated with Coffee Intake:

1. Excessive use can lead to dependence. Withdrawal symptoms including headaches may develop if you stop drinking it.

2. Decreases the absorption of iron and calcium.

3. Boiled coffee contains compounds that increase LDL cholesterol levels. Filtered and unfiltered coffee raises plasma homocysteine levels; both of which are associated with heart disease.

4. Coffee can contribute to high blood pressure and irregular heartbeats.

5. It is a mild diuretic and can cause dehydration.

6. Excessive consumption of coffee as a stimulant when you should be resting can lead to a worsening of fatigue.

7. If your liver cannot process the caffeine effectively, side effects such as feeling jittery or having an inability to sleep can worsen.

8. If the coffee is not organic then you are increasing your exposure to pesticides.

References:

1. Saaksjarvi K, Knekt P, et al. Prospective study of coffee consumption and risk of Parkinson's disease. PubMed

2. Hu G, Bidel S, Jousilahti P, et al. Coffee and tea consumption and the risk of Parkinson's disease. PubMed

3. van Dam RM, Willett WC, et al. Coffee, caffeine, and risk of type 2 diabetes: a prospective cohort study in younger and middle-aged U.S. women. Diabetes Care. PubMed

4. Leitzmann MF, Stampfer MJ, et al. Coffee intake is associated with lower risk of symptomatic gallstone disease in women. Gastroenterology. PubMed

5. Arendash GW, Schleif W, et al. Caffeine protects Alzheimer's mice against cognitive impairment and reduces brain beta-amyloid production. Neuroscience. PubMed

6. Urgert R, Essed N, et al. Separate effects of the coffee diterpenes cafestol and kahweol on serum lipids and liver aminotransferases. PubMed

7. Urgert R, Weusten-van der Wouw MP, et al. Chronic consumers of boiled coffee have elevated serum levels of lipoprotein(a). PubMed

8. Winkelmayer WC, Stampfer MJ, et al. Habitual caffeine intake and the risk of hypertension in women. PubMed

9. Hallstrom H, Wolk A, et al. Coffee, tea and caffeine consumption in relation to osteoporotic fracture risk in a cohort of Swedish women. PubMed

10. Wu, Jiang-nan; Ho, Suzanne C; et al. (2009). "Coffee consumption and risk of coronary heart diseases: A meta-analysis of 21 prospective cohort studies". International Journal of Cardiology 137 (3): 216–25. doi:10.1016/j.ijcard.2008.06.051. PMID 18707777.

11. Mol Nutr Food Res. 2010 Dec; 54(12):1734-43. doi: 10.1002/mnfr.201000147. Antioxidant effectiveness of coffee extracts and selected constituents in cell-free systems and human colon cell lines. Bakuradze T, Lang R, et al. Department of Chemistry, Division of Food Chemistry and Toxicology, University of Kaiserslautern, Kaiserslautern, Germany.

12. Hepatology. 2010 Nov; 52(5):1652-61.Coffee reduces liver damage in a rat model of steatohepatitis: the underlying mechanisms and the role of polyphenols and melanoidins.

13. Vitaglione P, Morisco F, et al. Department of Food Science, University of Napoli Federico II, Portici, Italy. paola.vitaglione@unina.it

14. Mol Nutr Food Res. 2010 Dec;54(12):1722-33. doi: 10.1002/mnfr.201000048. Instant coffee with high chlorogenic acid levels protects humans against oxidative damage of macromolecules.

15. Hoelzl C, Knasmüller S, et al. Department of Medicine I, Institute of Cancer Research, Medical University of Vienna, Vienna, Austria.

16. Cochrane Database Syst Rev. 2010 Jan 20;(1):CD001112. Caffeine for asthma. Welsh EJ, Bara A, et al. Community Health Sciences, St George's, University of London, Cranmer Terrace, London, UK, SW17 0RE.

17. Textbook of Natural Medicine. Pizzorno and Murray 2nd ed. Churchhill Livingston

Blood Sugar

Sickly Sweet

In the body, all carbohydrates are broken down into sugar. When you eat foods high in carbohydrates, the body uses enzymes to break them down into their smallest usable components: glucose, fructose and galactose. The sugars are absorbed into the blood stream so they can be delivered to the body's cells for energy. Sugar cannot enter the cells to make energy without the help of insulin. Insulin is a hormone produced by the pancreas and is the key that unlocks the door allowing sugar into the cells. Type I diabetics have lost their ability to make their own insulin. Without insulin injections they cannot survive because their cells will starve.

The body tightly regulates blood sugar. When blood sugar is too low, a hormone (glucagon) signals the liver to release sugar stored in the form of glycogen while adrenaline is secreted to increase appetite, mobilize stored sugar and motivate us to eat. The brain is completely dependent on sugar for fuel. In hypoglycemia, these hormones (glucagon and adrenaline) are released to protect the brain and tell your body to find an energy source fast. In contrast, if your blood sugar is too high then insulin is released to mobilize sugar into cells and store the excess as glycogen or in fat stores.

Unfortunately, this controlled process can go 'terribly' wrong. A diet high in carbohydrates places additional stress on the system resulting in the over secretion of insulin. Excess amounts of insulin rapidly lowers blood sugar and causes symptoms of hypoglycemia including dizziness, nausea, fatigue, irritability, hunger and headaches. In severe situations, seizures, coma and death can result which are associated with over-injecting insulin in diabetics.

Over time increased insulin levels promote weight gain and insulin resistance. In the case of insulin resistance, the cells become desensitized to insulin, requiring additional amounts from the pancreas to achieve the same effect. Eventually the overworked pancreas leads to Type II diabetes as the blood sugar constantly remains elevated and therefore unable to enter the cells. Uncontrolled blood sugar results in widespread damage over time. Blood vessels become sugar coated causing damage to the eyes, kidneys and cardiovascular system.

Glycemic Index & Glycemic Load

The type of carbohydrates you eat can have an effect on your blood sugar. Some foods are broken down more slowly and have a more gradual effect on the blood sugar. Those are foods typically higher in fiber like beans or higher in fat like dairy. Usually refined foods like white pasta or bread require very little effort to break down and blood sugar rises rapidly. The glycemic index grades foods based on how fast they increase blood sugar levels. Foods high on the glycemic index rapidly raise blood sugar levels and low glycemic foods do not. On the glycemic index anything scoring 55 or lower is considered a low glycemic food, while anything scoring 70 or above is considered high on the glycemic index. The glycemic load then takes the glycemic index and multiplies it by the quantity of the carbohydrates in the food. This gives a more accurate prediction of how high the blood sugar will rise after eating a certain food. A glycemic load of less than 10 is considered low while more than 20 is considered high.

Food	Glycemic Index High >70, Low<55 (good)	Serving Size (g)	Glycemic Load High >20, Low <10 (good)
Candy/Sweets			
Snickers	68	60g (1/2 bar)	23
Honey	87	2 Tbsp.	17.9
Table sugar	68	2 Tsps.	7
Peanut M&Ms	33	30g (1 oz.)	5.6
Dark chocolate	23	37g (1 oz.)	4.4
Breads & Cereals			
Bagel	72	89g (1/4 in.)	33
Corn bread	110	60g (1 piece)	30.8
Corn Chex	83	30g (1 cup)	20.8
Cheerios	74	30g (1 cup)	13.3
Rye Bread, 100%	65	32g (1 slice)	8.5
Corn Tortilla	70	24g (1 tortilla)	7.7
Popcorn	55	8g (1 cup)	2.8
Beverages			
Cola, carbonated	63	370g (12oz can)	25.2
Cranberry cocktail	68	253g (1 cup)	24.5
Orange juice	57	249g (1 cup)	14.25
Tomato juice	38	243g (1 cup)	3.4
Legumes			
Chickpeas	31	240g (1 cup)	13.3
Kidney beans	27	256g (1 cup)	7
Lentils	29	198g (1 cup)	7
Peanuts	13	146g (1 cup)	1.6
Vegetables			
Yellow Corn	55	166g (1 cup)	61.5
Potato	104	213g (1 med)	36.4
Tomato	38	123g (1 med)	1.5
Broccoli, cooked	0	78g (1/2 cup)	0

Spinach	0	30g (1 cup)	0
Fruit			
Raisins	64	43g (small box)	20.5
Banana	51	118g (1 med)	12.2
Watermelon	72	152g (1 cup)	7.2
Grapes	43	92g (1 cup)	6.5
Peach	28	98g (1 med)	2.2
Dairy			
Ice Cream (low fat)	47	76g (1/2 cup)	9.4
Yogurt, plain	36	245g (1 cup)	6.1

Please see http://www.mendosa.com/gilists.htm for a more comprehensive list. **Note**: Although a particular food may have a low Glycemic index or load, keep in mind the number of calories in a serving.

References:
1. T B. Nutritional biochemistry. Academic Pr; 1999
2. AR G. Nutritional Medicine. Concord NH: Fritz Perlberg Publishing; 2011
3. JE P, MT M. Textbook of natural medicine. Churchill Livingstone; 2006
4. R T. The glycemic-load diet: A powerful new program for losing weight and reversing insulin resistance. McGraw-Hill; 2006

Pop

More than just bubbles

Soda pop was once an occasional treat contained in a tiny glass bottle. It now comes in bucket sizes and is a staple item in many people's diet. There are countless varieties and methods of sweetening, preserving and coloring soft drinks. From high fructose corn syrup to aspartame, there are many troubling issues that come with the overconsumption of pop.

1. High Fructose Corn Syrup: can cause insulin resistance and weight gain (over time obesity and diabetes), high cholesterol and triglycerides along with increased oxidation, (over time heart disease). Oxidation is the reason we take anti-oxidants. Mercury is used in the processing of HFCS and therefore there is possible mercury exposure. HFCS does not make you feel full, resulting in overconsumption *(please refer to Heavy Metals for more information)*.

2. Artificial Sweeteners: aspartame, acesulfame-potassium and neotame can cause headaches, mental confusion, depression, liver effects, kidney effects, bronchitis, loss of appetite, nausea, lack of balance, visual disturbances, numbness, memory loss, severe mood swings, suicidal tendencies, weight gain and can possibly cause cancer. Sucralose can cause reactions such as headaches. There are currently no long-term human studies on its safety available for public review.

3. Brominated Vegetable Oil (BVO): is found in cloudy looking drinks like yellow sodas. This substance is banned in many European countries and has been reported to cause serious toxicity with overconsumption such as headaches, fatigue, memory loss, loss of coordination, rashes, irritability, psychosis, confusion and hallucinations.

4. Phosphoric Acid: is found in many soft drinks in particular the colas. Can reduce bone mineral density by upsetting the calcium phosphorus balance contributing significantly to osteopenia or osteoporosis.

5. Sodium Benzoate and Artificial Coloring: a preservative found in many soft drinks, it has been known to cause asthma attacks and behavioral changes in sensitive people.

References:

1. Abdelmalek, M.F., A. Suzuki et al. "Increased Fructose Consumption is Associated With Fibrosis Severity in Patients With Nonalcoholic Fatty Liver Disease." Hepatology 51.6 (2010): 1961-71

2. Bateman, B., JO Warner et al. "The Effects of a Double Blind, Placebo Controlled, Artificial Food Colourings and Benzoate Preservative Challenge on Hyperactivity in a General Population Sample of Preschool Children." Archives of Disease in Childhood 89.6 (2004): 506.

3. Horowitz, B.Z. "Bromism From Excessive Cola Consumption." Clinical Toxicology 35.3 (1997): 315-20.

4. Ludwig, D.S., K.E. Peterson, and S.L. Gortmaker. "Relation Between Consumption of Sugar-Sweetened Drinks and Childhood Obesity: A Prospective, Observational Analysis." The Lancet 357.9255 (2001): 505-08.

5. Maher, T.J., and R.J. Wurtman. "Possible Neurologic Effects of Aspartame, a Widely Used Food Additive." Environmental Health Perspectives 75 (1987): 53.

6. McGartland, C., PJ Robson et al. "Carbonated Soft Drink Consumption and Bone Mineral Density in Adolescence: The Northern Ireland Young Hearts Project." Journal of bone and mineral research 18.9 (2003): 1563-69.

7. Mercola, J., and K.D. Pearsall. "Sweet Deception: Why Splenda®, Nutrasweet®, and the Fda May be Hazardous to Your Health." (2007)

8. Oney, J.W., N.B. Farber et al. "Increasing Brain Tumor Rates: Is There a Link to Aspartame?" Journal of Neuropathology & Experimental Neurology 55.11 (1996): 1115.

9. Shoham, D.A., R. Durazo-Arvizu et al. "Sugary Soda Consumption and Albuminuria: Results From the National Health and Nutrition Examination Survey, 1999–2004." PLoS One 3.10 (2008): e3431.

10. Tsakiris, S., A. Giannoulia-Karantana et al. "The Effect of Aspartame Metabolites on Human Erythrocyte Membrane Acetylcholinesterase Activity." Pharmacological research 53.1 (2006): 1-5.

11. Tucker, K.L., K. Morita et al. "Colas, But Not Other Carbonated Beverages, Are Associated With Low Bone Mineral Density in Older Women: The Framingham Osteoporosis Study." The American journal of clinical nutrition 84.4 (2006): 936.

12. Van den Eeden, SK, TD Koepsell et al. "Aspartame Ingestion and Headaches: A Randomized Crossover Trial." Neurology 44.10 (1994): 1787.

13. Ogur, R., B. Uysal et al. "Evaluation of the Effect of Cola Drinks on Bone Mineral Density and Associated Factors." Basic & clinical pharmacology & toxicology 100.5 (2007): 334-38.

Smoking

A lethal kiss

The strong medical evidence relating tobacco smoke to very serious health problems is difficult to ignore. Today, smoking tobacco is the leading cause of preventable death in Canada. The detrimental health impacts are observed by all ages from unborn babies to seniors. Tobacco is responsible for the death of more than five million people worldwide every year. The World Health Organization (WHO) believes that, if current trends continue, more than eight million people will die from tobacco use per year by 2030 and one billion people in the entire 21st century.

Research has clearly demonstrated that people with repeated exposure to tobacco smoke are most likely to develop and die from heart problems, lung cancer and respiratory difficulties. There are more than 4,000 chemicals in tobacco smoke, including the heavy metals cadmium and arsenic *(please refer to Heavy Metals for more information)*. More than 50 of these chemicals are known carcinogens. In Canada, lung cancer is the leading cause of death with tobacco smoke accounting for 85% of all new cases. Smoking can lead to genetic alterations in lung cells. Respiratory symptoms including coughing, phlegm, wheezing and labored breathing are just some of the early changes that can result. Asthmatic bronchitis, chronic bronchitis and emphysema are Chronic Obstructive Pulmonary Diseases that can be attributed to the chemicals found in tobacco smoke.

Digestive and other respiratory cancers, specifically mouth, throat, esophageal, stomach and pancreatic have been correlated with smoking tobacco. There is also an increased risk of developing leukemia, bladder and kidney cancer. Females especially, should be concerned about the higher risk of cervical cancer.

Smoking inhibits the flow of blood throughout the body resulting in the blockage of arteries and injuries to blood vessels of the heart, brain and extremities. Cardiovascular disease, angina, coronary heart disease and heart attacks can also be caused by smoking. Peripheral vascular disease (blockages in the circulation to the legs) and impotence can occur. Cerebrovascular disease including the risk of stroke is 50% higher in smokers. This risk is greatly elevated by the number of cigarettes smoked per day. Interestingly, the risk of stroke is reduced by about 50% within one year of smoking cessation and can return to the same level as those who have never smoked within five years.

Surprisingly, second hand smoke can lead to just as many health concerns. According to the WHO, it is responsible for about 600,000 deaths per year and about 1% of the global burden of disease worldwide. As children breathe faster than adults and require twice the amount of oxygen, they are especially vulnerable to environmental tobacco smoke. Toxins ingested circulate twice as fast in their bodies. The blood brain barrier that prevents harmful substances from entering the brain is not as developed, allowing easier accessibility for many drugs and toxins. Children are therefore more likely to develop ear infections, throat irritations and excessive coughing; their chances of developing asthma increases by 200 to 400 percent. Unfortunately, the adverse effects of smoking extend well beyond the individual smoker.

Virtually every organ in the body is negatively affected by tobacco. The strong evidence correlating smoke to the development of disease should be advertised and considered by all ages of the population. At NaturoMedic.com, we believe that the adverse effects of smoking can directly impact your health and your therapeutic treatments. We recommend that you should reduce smoking, work towards quitting smoking and avoid environments where you are exposed to smoke.

References:
1. Health Canada: http://www.hc-sc.gc.ca/hc-ps/tobac-tabac/research-recherche/stat/_ctums-_esutc_2000/yanosc-vesfcc-eng.php
2. World Health Organization:
    http://www.who.int/gho/phe/secondhand_smoke/en/

Downloadable Books:

Canadian Cancer Society:

One Step at a Time: for smokers who don't want to quit

http://www.cancer.ca/Canada-wide/Publications/Alphabetical%20list%20of%20publications/~/media/CCS/Canada%20wide/Files%20List/English%20files%20heading/Library%20PDFs%20-%20English/osaat-dont_want_to_quit_en_nov2009.ashx

One Step at a Time: for smokers who want to quit

http://www.cancer.ca/Canada-wide/Publications/Alphabetical%20list%20of%20publications/~/media/CCS/Canada%20wide/Files%20List/English%20files%20heading/Library%20PDFs%20-%20English/osaat-want_to_quit_en_nov2009.ashx

Street Drugs

A Road to Nowhere

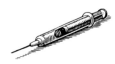 Drug usage for pleasure has been a common practice for thousands of years and is well documented throughout history. Egyptians used wine, narcotics were consumed as early as 4000 B.C. and marijuana was applied medicinally in 2737 BC China. A desire to consume substances that enhance relaxation, invoke stimulation or create euphoria has always existed.

Opium is a prime example of a highly addictive drug introduced early on in human history. Originally from the poppy plant, this drug was used primarily for treating pain, although it was also liberally used for any ailment ranging from coughs to diarrhea. The use of opium spread from Asia to the West, peaking in the 19th century. A variety of stronger painkillers, such as morphine, were eventually isolated from the opium poppy. During the American Civil War, morphine was used freely and wounded veterans returned home with their kits of morphine. Cocaine and heroin were sold as patent medicines in the 19th and early 20th centuries and marketed as treatments for a wide variety of ailments. By the early 1900s there were an estimated 250,000 addicts in the United States. Due to their addictive properties, strict laws prohibiting their use were developed. In 1908, Canada prohibited the import, manufacturing and sale of opium, the first Western nation to do so. Even with these laws, illegal drugs are still produced from morphine, such as heroin which causes major harm in terms of addiction and the resulting crime associated with illegal drug use.

Addictive drugs work by increasing the chemical dopamine that stimulates the pleasure center of the brain. Initially there is a feeling of euphoria, however with continual use, the drug actually changes the chemistry of the brain, requiring larger amounts of the drug to produce the same effect. This is known as tolerance. When people rely on the drug to feel normal they have developed physical dependence. At that point, many are willing to do whatever it takes to get their next "fix", including engaging in risky behavior and crime, in order to avoid any withdrawal symptoms. During periods of withdrawal, other physical symptoms can develop including muscle and bone pain, insomnia, restlessness, diarrhea and vomiting, cold flashes, involuntary tremors and much more.

Top Ten Street (Recreational) Drugs

- Solvents (gasoline huffing)
- Benzodiazepines and barbituates
- Opium and opiates
- Heroin
- Cannabis (marijuana)
- Ecstasy (MDMA)
- LSD (aka acid)
- Amphetamines
- Mushrooms
- Cocaine

While there are many different street drugs being used, all have the potential to cause harm to your health with many having life-threatening consequences. Each drug often has specific side effects. Some of the common ones experienced are: blood shot eyes, dilated pupils, blurred vision, increased body temperature, heart rate and blood pressure, nausea, abdominal pain, headaches, chills, sweating, muscle cramping and tremors. The life-threatening outcomes may also vary by dosage and intensity of the drug. These include changes in heart rhythm, heart attacks, respiratory failure, strokes, seizures and even death.

The dangers to your body and the warnings against addictive street drugs are something we have all heard throughout the years. There are many resources and centers available for drug rehabilitation. It is also important to properly detoxify these drugs from your system and support the body as it attempts to regain control over its necessary functions (*please refer to Detoxification for more information*). The long-term consequences of street drug use and addiction should not be easily dismissed. IV vitamins and minerals have proven to be very effective in healing the body and brain from substance abuse (*please refer to Intravenous Myers Cocktail for more information*).

References:
1. http://www.drug-rehabs.org/drughistory.php
2. http://uga-cdd.org/background.php
3. http://www.thecanadianencyclopedia.com/index.cfm?PgNm=TCE&Params=A1ARTA0002402

Choices

Diet and Food Allergies

The food selections we make have an important impact on health. The phrase that "you are what you eat" continues to be an accurate statement. The idea that food affects one's health and state of mind originated in 1800s with the philosopher Ludwig Feuerbach and the epicurean Anthelme Brillat-Savarin. The health status of cultures consuming a diet similar to their ancestors continues to exceed industrialized regions. In the 1930s, Dr. Weston Price observed the prevalence of disease and structural changes in societies with a diet of predominantly highly refined foods. Victor Lindlahr declared in 1940 that food controls health. He further stated that "ninety percent of the diseases known to man are caused by cheap foodstuffs." As these conclusions persisted, it became well-accepted that dietary changes can prevent, delay or treat chronic diseases. Nutrition can influence genetic expression and switch genes on and off, directly correlating to the literal meaning of "you are what you eat". The following sections introduce the most harmful aspects of the modern diet and their influences on health.

Refined Sugar

It is estimated that North Americans consume on average over 140-150 lbs. (64-68 kg) of refined sugar a year. Some eat closer to 200 lbs. (91 kg) and others much less (less than 50 lbs. /23 kg). This shocking amount has grown exponentially since 1905 when the average was only 5 lbs. (2 kg). The prevalent trend of diabetes and obesity should therefore not come as a surprise.

Sweetened drinks, especially pop, energy drinks and specialty coffees can account for a large component of your sugar source (*please refer to the individual sections for more information*). Sugar, among its many forms, is a main ingredient in pre-packaged food. Apart from its sweetening role it is also used as a preservative. Sugar at concentrations of 55-65% (i.e. jam) can prevent the growth of bacteria. Table sugar produced from sugar cane or beets no longer has the benefit of the original plant. The fiber, vitamins, minerals and enzymes used for digestion are extracted during the manufacturing process. The concentrated sugar, refined of its natural ingredients results in insulin spikes, hypoglycemia and insulin resistance with continual consumption. Uncontrolled blood sugar and insulin levels are two major factors in many chronic diseases including heart disease, diabetes, cancer, obesity, arthritis and immune dysfunction (*please refer to Blood Sugar for more information)*. Additionally, daily sugar consumption can lead to decreased energy, anxiety, fatigue, bloating, migraines, high blood pressure and eczema, etc.

Corn sweeteners account for an estimated 40-80 lbs. (18-36 kg) of the 150 lbs. (68 kg) of consumed sugar. The common use of high fructose corn syrup (HFCS) began in the 1970's with the high taxes (tariffs) placed on importing sugar into North America. Consequently, the rate of obese or overweight children and teens has increased by 100%. Mercury is a toxic heavy metal used in the manufacturing process of HFCS and theoretically should be removed from the final product. Research has determined that a portion of the highly processed sweetener has been contaminated. In 2003, 79% of the total mercury used in production could not be accounted for (equivalent to 30 out of 38 tons/3,000 kg out of 3,800 kg). Samples from 55 foods found detectable levels of mercury in 31% of items.

The U.S. Environment Protection Agency recommends a maximum ingestion of 5.5 µg/day of mercury for the average American woman of childbearing age. If a can of cola has 39 g of HFCS then it could contain as much as 22.23 µg of mercury. This well exceeds the accepted safe amount. Mercury is very toxic to the brain, immune system, kidneys and lungs (*please refer to Heavy Metals for more information*). The heavy metal is not quite what you bargained for when you purchased your soda. Remember to read labels and pay attention to the sugar content.

Flour
Flour is a staple in most North American diets. The average Canadian consumes 43.7 kg (96 lbs.) of wheat flour per year. Modern flour is very different than 200 years ago. Traditionally, the inedible shell was removed from the grain and the remainder was consumed: the bran (the outside of the grain; a good source of fiber), the germ (a little pocket on the inside of the grain; a good source of nutrients and anti-oxidants) and the endosperm (most of the inside of the grain: made up of starch). Today the refined flour is merely the endosperm. Although, enriched flour contains synthetic vitamins but no minerals or fiber.

Refined flour does not appeal to microorganisms and does not spoil. It has a long shelf life and can be shipped without refrigeration. Similar to sugar, once stripped of many nutritional components, the quick metabolism of flour by the body also leads to spikes in blood sugar and insulin. This consequently, results in many of the same health concerns.

North American wheat is not equivalent to wheat grown in more temperate European climates. The two strains here, Marquis and Durham semolina, have been adapted to withstand Prairie weather and yield maximum crop. European bread is often more tolerable to the digestive system. Gluten is usually the culprit of many digestive difficulties.

Gluten is the protein found in wheat. Today, 1 in 133 people are diagnosed with celiac disease in Canada. This is a genetic disease that results in destruction of the lining of the gut when exposed to gluten. In addition to celiac, 1 in 3 Canadians cannot tolerate large amounts of gluten without having symptoms of gas, bloating and abdominal pain. Rotating grains or simply switching to another grain like spelt or rye may alleviate wheat sensitivities (not an option for celiac sufferers).

Salt

Salt is highly valued as a commodity worldwide and was historically used as a preservative. Concentrations greater than 10% will inhibit the growth of most microorganisms. Salt (sodium chloride) is another major ingredient of processed foods. North Americans consume 12-27g of sodium a day. The total daily intake is often comprised of 50% from processed foods and condiments, 45% from additional salt during consumption and only 5% occurring naturally in food.

Along with the mineral electrolytes, calcium, potassium, magnesium and chloride, salt is a necessary part of the diet. A proper balance should be maintained to prevent health complications. Fruits and vegetables are good sources of electrolytes, whereas processed foods contain sodium chloride and are void of potassium and magnesium. Salt is the common culprit of elevated blood pressure and fluid retention. Unbalanced electrolytes (high salts with low magnesium, potassium and calcium) have also been shown to aggravate migraines, PMS and contribute to cancer.

Fat

Fat is commonly added to premade or processed foods. Prior to 1910, butterfat, beef tallow and lard were the primary fats found in foods. The ability to make oil byproducts, (i.e. soybean oil) into a solid state (i.e. butter or lard) forever changed food. As a result of the cost saving advantages, hydrogenated oils are now the main sources of fat in processed foods. These include margarine, peanut butter and bakery products.

The negative health effects of **hydrogenated oils** are mainly due to trans-fatty acids. While fat is essential to life, many consume more bad fats than good fats (i.e. omega-3 fatty acids). Trans-fatty acids do occur naturally in animal products, meat and dairy, though they make up only 2-5% of the total fat. Adversely, in processed food trans-fat can account for 50-60% of the total fat. Unlike a healthy fat, when trans-fat incorporates into our body tissue they decrease HDL (High Density Lipoprotein, aka the "good cholesterol"), make blood sticky, increase the likelihood of a clot and elevate lipoprotein A (a marker for heart disease). Trans-

89

fatty acid also affects insulin, blood sugar, weight and the risk of diabetes. Breast milk containing high amounts of trans-fatty acids has also been shown to lower visual acuity in babies.

Heating vegetable oils, including olive oil, to high temperatures can form trans-fatty acids and destroy all health benefits. Use oil-less cooking methods or an oil that is more resistant to damage (i.e. coconut oil) or add your olive oil after cooking for flavor to prevent adding trans fats to your meals.

Dairy

In 2008, the average Canadian drank 57.7 L of milk. Milk was once a good nutritional source of vitamins, minerals and healthy fats. The raw milk still contained its natural enzymes for digestion. Cows roamed and grazed on natural organic grass fields. The dairy industry today is very different. The majority of milk produced in North America is pasteurized and homogenized. Vitamins and enzymes are destroyed as the milk is heated to kill microorganisms.

Pasteurization is the process of heating a liquid to a high temperature to sterilize it. With milk, heating alters the molecular configuration of casein (milk protein) into a gastrointestinal irritant, preventing our ability to absorb calcium. An increase in heart disease has actually been associated with the introduction of pasteurized milk. Cultures where milk is fermented instead of pasteurized have essentially no heart disease.

The invention of **homogenization** has been referred to as the "worst thing that dairymen did to milk" (Homogenized Milk: Rocket Fuel for Cancer by Robert Cohen, Executive Director of the Dairy Education Board). Milk is pushed through a fine filter at pressures of 4,000 pounds per square inch. The fat globules are made at least 10 times smaller and become evenly dispersed throughout the milk, allowing them to bypass digestion. Proteins and enzymes are not metabolized and enter the bloodstream. These surviving substances attack arterial walls, forcing the body to protect itself with cholesterol and leading to heart disease. Cardiologists discovered that an enzyme from milk, bovine xanthene oxidase, negatively affects victims of heart attacks. Children are even showing signs of hardened arteries.

Homogenization disrupts digestive processes stimulating the body to produce histamine and mucous in response to foreign proteins. Certain milk proteins are also similar to human proteins and therefore can trigger autoimmune reactions (via a process called cross reactivity).

Remnants of **antibiotics** in milk also contribute to dairy's ill effects. There are at least 52 known antibiotics used to treat infections in cows and only 30 approved by the FDA. Residues of antibiotics can remain in the cow's milk for at least 4 to

7 milkings following antibiotic cessation. This milk should technically be disposed of, although this is not always the case. The milk from a single cow on antibiotics can contaminate an entire truck load of milk. The drug residues in milk contribute to antibiotic resistance and allergic reactions. Dairy products are also a concentrated source of **pesticides and herbicides**. When cows are fed heavily sprayed grains, the toxins become stored in fat and subsequently contaminate the milk (*please refer to Pesticides for more information*).

There are over 25 proteins in milk that can cause allergic reactions. The milk protein **casein** is one of the main causal factors for allergic reactions among dairy containing food. In general, milk increases mucus production and contributes to sinusitis, arthritis, allergies, ear infections, headaches, congestion, eczema, fatigue, asthma, colic and bed wetting in children. Dairy has also been implicated as a cause of Type I diabetes in children.

The milk sugar, **lactose**, presents another reason to question milks' health benefits. Over 7 million Canadians (20%) cannot digest the milk sugar lactose and the intolerance is a worldwide phenomenon. The ability to produce the necessary enzyme lactase for lactose digestion is typically lost after being weaned off breast milk. Without this enzyme, milk consumers can experience severe cramps, diarrhea, bloating and gas. Worldwide, there are differences in lactose intolerance that are dependent on the region's history of dairy farming. North West Europe and Scandinavia have only a 3-8% prevalence of lactose intolerance and are therefore more able to digest the milk sugar. South Eastern Asia is 100% intolerant to lactose. Throughout Europe, the amount rises to 70% the closer you live to Southern Italy and Turkey. Africa (except for cattle raising nomads), Asia and South America have a prevalence of 50%. Finally, 90% of Native Americans are lactose intolerant. Basically, two thirds of the world's population is unable to digest lactose.

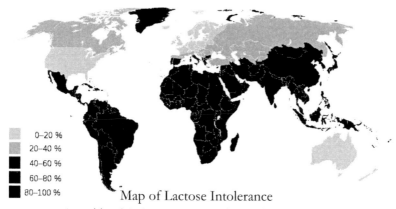

0–20 %
20–40 %
40–60 %
60–80 %
80–100 %

Map of Lactose Intolerance
http://eatdahplant.tumblr.com/image/5736643988

Processed Foods

The ability of processed foods to survive in vending machines while still looking palatable is largely due to colorings and additives. The FDA has approved over 2800 **food additives** and it is estimated that the average person consumes 13-15 g per day. Some additives are natural and have health promoting properties and others have known side effects. For example, vitamin E or C can be used in preservation but the colouring agent tartrazine commonly causes reactions especially in children (i.e. asthma and hives). Tartrazine and benzoate (other food additives) increase histamine producing mast cells and the likelihood of developing allergies, asthma and eczema. Sulfites, another common preservative found in pickled foods, dried fruit, wine and wine vinegars, can lead to severe reactions of asthma, hives and life threatening anaphylactic shock. MSG is added to many soups, dressings, frozen foods and snack foods to add flavor yet it can often cause palpitations, headaches, abdominal pain and urinary urgency. Making your own food is the safest way to ensure that you avoid additives. Always remember to read labels.

In **summary**, the modern diet is somewhat lacking in regards to nutritional and beneficial substances. Making changes to the diet is not easy and impossible to do overnight. There are many considerations that affect healthy eating which should be addressed: cooking for one or a family, time, finances, product availability, organic foods *(please refer to Pesticides for more information)*, recipe knowledge, desire to cook, food preferences, food allergies and finally, religious or cultural beliefs. The challenges can seem daunting at first, but with determination everyone can persevere. Begin slowly and eventually the small steps will make the difference *(please refer to Changing Habits for more information)*.

Food Allergies

Not only do we have challenges with nutritional aspects of our food, we can also have individual reactions to healthy food. Many nutrient rich foods cannot be freely consumed without consequences. There are several forms of allergies and intolerances. Moreover, there is a difference between an allergy and sensitivity to food. **Allergies** are often narrowly defined as an inappropriate immune response to an allergen, which can range from a mild to severe reaction. This refers to an anaphylactic response to nuts, eggs, seafood, strawberries etc. and common triggers seen on standard allergy tests. **Food sensitivities/intolerance**, on the other hand, encompasses a broader definition and rarely appear on typical tests. Most of the population suffers from food intolerances which denote an inappropriate functional response to an allergen causing symptoms of fatigue, headaches, joint pain, abdominal discomfort, digestive complaints or recurring infections. The modern diet is a gateway for toxins, harmful substances, highly refined food, malnutrition, allergies and food intolerances. It is no surprising that diet maintains an influential role in health and growing disease trends.

To help determine which food items are important to eliminate we have included a list of common allergy tests employed by numerous practitioners. We have also listed a variety of effective therapies NaturoMedic.com has used to reverse symptoms and improve health (*please refer to the specific chapter for more information on the therapy*).

Common Testing for Allergies

Allergy Test	How it's Performed	What it's good for testing
ELISA	Take a blood sample and test to see if there is an immune response (IgG & IgE antibodies stick to allergen) when mixed with different allergens.	Food and environmental allergies where there is an immune response. Works only for foods that have been recently ingested.
RAST	Take a blood sample and add tagged allergens to the blood sample to see if there is an immune response (IgE antibodies stick to allergen).	Food and environmental allergies of a specific sort (IgE antibody reactions). Good for inhalants not very sensitive for foods.
Skin prick test	Small needles are used to prick the skin and introduce an allergen to see if there is a specific reaction (redness and swelling at the site)	Food and environmental allergies of a specific sort (IgE antibody reactions in the skin) better for inhalants than food.
Skin patch test	Patches covered with suspected allergen are taped onto skin and left in place for 48 hours to see if a rash forms at site of patch	Used to test for substances that are irritating to the skin through contact like chemicals or other things in the environment.
Intradermal test	Allergen in solution is injected into the skin to see if there is a specific reaction at the site (redness and swelling)	Used mostly to test for reactions to insect venom and penicillin.
Elimination Diet	A diet where the most common allergic foods are eliminated for a period of time and then reintroduced 1 at a time to note any reactions.	Used to find common food sensitivities. They could be foods that cause an immune reaction or other symptoms.
Provocation Testing	Also called a challenge test. Escalating amounts of the allergen are usually given by mouth or inhaled over a period of time to see if there are any immediate or delayed reactions occur.	Used to find immediate or delayed responses to foods or inhaled allergens. A very time consuming procedure done in an allergist's office.

Electrodermal testing	Using various computer systems to measure energy changes at acupuncture points as the body is exposed to different allergens.	Used to find allergies or sensitivities to foods and environmental allergies. Not dependent on an immune response.
Muscle Testing	Using the principles of applied kinesiology a patients is tested for various symptoms.	Used to find allergies or sensitivities to any food or substance even if the symptoms are not an immune response.

Therapies offered to help with Food allergies and sensitivities:

- Eliminate Allergy Technique
- Cleansing Diet
- Fasting
- Homeopathy
- Nutritional Supplements

References:

1. RM, W. What's Milk Got? Townsend Letter for Doctors & Patients 128-130 (2002).
2. D, W., J, S., et al. Not So Sweet: Missing Mercury and High Fructose Corn Syrup. (2009).
3. AN, S. Nutritionally Incorrect: Why the Modern Diet is Dangerous and How to Defend Yourself. (Woodland Publishing, Pleasant Grove, 2002).
4. A, S. & T, M. The Whole Life Nutrition Cookbook (Whole Life Press, Bellingham, WA, 2008).
5. WA, P. Nutrition and Physical Degeneration (Price-Pottenger Nutrition Foundation, La Mesa, 2008).
6. Pizzorno, J. & Murray, M. Textbook of Natural Medicine (Churchill Livingston, St Louis, 2006).
7. Luck, E., Jaeger, M. & Lichen, S. F. Antimicrobial food additives: characteristics, uses, effects (Springer Verilog, 1997).
8. Gaby. Nutritional Medicine 2011
9. Enid, M. G. Know Your Fats : The Complete Primer for Understanding the Nutrition of Fats, Oils and Cholesterol (Bethesda PR, 2000).
10. http://www.statcan.gc.ca/ads-annonces/23f0001x/hl-fs-eng.htm#a4
11. http://www4.agr.gc.ca/AAFC-AAC/display-afficher.do?id=1286909778024&lang=eng
12. http://www.cdhf.ca/digestive-disorders/statistics.shtml
13. http://www.foodreactions.org/intolerance/lactose/prevalence.htm
14. Atkins, D. Food allergy: diagnosis and management. Prim Care 35, 119-40, vii (2008).

15. AW, B. & HA, S. Diagnostic approaches to the patient with suspected food allergies*. The Journal of Pediatrics 121, S64-S71 (1992).

16. TJ, D. Unorthodox allergy procedures. Archives Of Disease In Childhood 62, 1060-1062 (1987).

17. K, E. & H, M. Chronisch-entzundliche Darmerkrankungen (Colitis ulcerosa; Enteritis regionalis Crohn): Atiologie und Therapieergebnisse unter Anwendung der bioenergetischen Funktionsdiagnostik und der Magnetfrequenzakupunktur. Forschende Komplementarmedizin 5, 178-182 (1998).

18. Fleischer, D. M. & Atkins, D. Evaluation of the patient with suspected eosinophilic gastrointestinal disease. Immunol Allergy Clin North Am 29, 53-63, ix (2009).

19. K, K. Clinical outcomes of a diagnostic and treatment protocol in allergy/sensitivity patients. Alternative Medicine Review 6, 188-202 (2001).

20. R, L. Ending allergies with acupuncture. Nambudripad Allergy Elimination Technique (NAET). Alternative Medicine Magazine Jan, 58-61 (1999).

21. X, L. Complementary and alternative medicine in pediatric allergic disorders. Current Opinion in Allergy & Clinical Immunology 9, 161-167 (2009).

22. KJ, M. Allergiebehandlung mit Bioresonanz-Therapie - mehr als Hoffnung: Heilung! Erfahrungsheilkunde 48, 309-316 (1999).

23. Pfab F, et al. Influence of acupuncture on type I hypersensitivity itch and the wheal and flare response in adults with atopic eczema - a blinded, randomized, placebo- controlled, crossover trial. Allergy 65, 903-910 (2009).

24. L, R. & JV, W. What's Really Making You Sick? Life Extension Magazine (2010).

25. Salvatori, N. et al. Asthma induced by inhalation of flour in adults with food allergy to wheat. Clin Exp Allergy 38, 1349-1356 (2008).

26. H, S. 9. Food allergy. Journal of Allergy and Clinical Immunology 111, 540-547 (2003).

27. HA, S. & DD, M. Food Allergies. JAMA 268, 2840-2844 (1992).

28. HA, S. Food allergy. Part 2: Diagnosis and management. The Journal of Allergy and Clinical Immunology 103, 981-989 (1999).

29. Schmitt WA, G, L. Muscle Testing Findings with Serum Immunologobulin Levels for Food Allergies. International Journal of Neuroscience 96, 237-244 (1998).

30. C, W. Food Allergies. Oriental Medicine Journal 15, 14-15 (2007).

31. http://www.forbes.com/sites/sap/2012/10/09/nutrigenomics-the-study-of-you-are-what-you-eat/

32. http://www.naturalnews.com/022967_milk_pasteurization_dairy.html#ixzz2M0rXXkUX

33. Cohen, R. Homegenized Milk: Rocket Fuel For Cancer. http://health101.org/art_milk_cancer_fuel.htm

Vitamin and Mineral Deficiencies

Nutrient Essentials

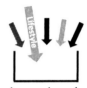

Vitamins

Vitamins are organic substances that your body needs for normal growth and development. They are necessary for health, general well-being and vitality. There are 13 essential vitamins required by your body that can be classified into two categories, fat soluble and water soluble. Fat soluble vitamins, A, D, E, and K, dissolve in fat and can be stored in the body for longer periods than water-soluble vitamins. Water soluble vitamins, C and the B vitamins, need to dissolve in water before being absorbed by the body. Any water soluble vitamin that cannot be stored passes through the urinary system and is lost. A fresh supply of these vitamins is therefore required daily. We have found that a lot of people have vitamin deficiencies. Interestingly, the greatest cause of these has not been from lack of exposure, but actually from sensitivity to the vitamin. These sensitivities can result in poor absorption, decreased energy, poor memory, headaches and multiple allergies. The Eliminate Allergy Technique (EAT) is an effective treatment for removing sensitivities (*please refer to EAT for more information*).

Minerals

Minerals are inorganic micronutrients required by the body to function optimally. There are 16 essential minerals that must be supplied by our diets. These minerals are divided into two groups: major and trace minerals. Major minerals, like calcium, chloride, magnesium, phosphorus, potassium, sodium and sulfur, are found in our body in amounts larger than 5 grams. Trace minerals, like chromium, copper, fluoride, iodine, iron, manganese, selenium and zinc, are found in our body in amounts less than 5 grams. Below is a list of important information about certain minerals that more commonly appear to be deficient in the population.

The following is a list of important vitamins (pg. 97-101) and minerals (pg.102-106) that are commonly found to be deficient in the population.

Vitamins

	What it does in the body	Symptoms of deficiency	Interactions with other nutrients	Foods high in nutrient	Interesting Facts
Water Soluble Vitamins					
Vitamin C	Collagen synthesis - important for skin and connective tissues. Important for immune function and detoxification	Severe deficiency (scurvy): bruising and bleeding problems, bone pain and osteoporosis, muscle pain, swelling, heart problems, fatigue and emotional changes. Some symptoms, especially cardiac can show up before someone is fully depleted	Carnitine is essential with vitamin C to make collagen. Vitamin C enhances absorption of iron. Vitamin E works with vitamin C in antioxidant function.	Citrus fruits, cantaloupe, broccoli, Brussels sprouts, cauliflower, potatoes	British sailors were referred to as limey's because they ate limes on their ships to avoid getting scurvy. Humans are one of the few mammals that cannot make vitamin C.
B1 (thiamine)	Important for energy production and making genetic building blocks (nucleic acids). Important to nerve function	Severe deficiency is called beriberi. Symptoms include weakness, weight loss, heart failure, swelling, peripheral neuropathy & psychiatric disturbances. Mild deficiency symptoms include fatigue, insomnia, loss of appetite, difficulties with memory and concentration. Deficiency can cause permanent damage and death.	Magnesium is needed to convert thiamine to its active form.	Whole grains, nuts, legumes, meat, and enriched flour	Significant amounts of thiamine are lost when cooking at high temperatures or in cooking water. Thiamine is required for alcohol metabolism, therefore alcoholics are significantly deficient in this nutrient.

97

Vitamins

	What it does in the body	Symptoms of deficiency	Interactions with other nutrients	Foods high in nutrient	Interesting Facts
Water Soluble Vitamins					
B5 (pantothenic acid)	Helps to produce and break down many important molecules in the body including fatty acids, proteins, brain chemicals, cholesterol and hemoglobin	Symptoms of deficiency include: burning sensation in the feet, numbness and tingling of the hands and feet, muscle weakness, recurrent colds or infections, stomach upset, dizziness with standing or bending over, low stomach acid, and depression	Some studies have shown that copper deficiency increases the requirements for B5	Meat, broccoli, avocados	Vitamin B5 is produced in the intestines by natural flora however the vitamin can also be destroyed by vinegar and baking soda
B6 pyridoxine	Plays a role in the immune system, helps break down proteins, sugars, and fats for energy, helps strengthen arterial walls	Symptoms of deficiency include: nervousness, depression, irritability, insomnia, confusion, inflamed tongue and mouth, abdominal pain, weakness, seizures, anemia, impaired immune function	B6 and magnesium work together, one helps the other get into our cells, Large doses of B6 increase the body's folate, and zinc requirements.	Potatoes, bananas, meat, poultry, fish and whole grains.	Riboflavin is needed to convert B6 to its active form, tongue and mouth symptoms from B2 might really be B6 deficiency

98

	What it does in the body	Symptoms of deficiency	Interactions with other nutrients	Foods high in nutrient	Interesting Facts
Water Soluble Vitamins					
Folate (folic acid)	Plays a role in DNA/RNA synthesis, involved in B12 metabolism, nervous system function, and immune system function	B12 deficiency is the best-known sign of folate deficiency. Symptoms include depression, anxiety, fatigue, apathy, confusion, or dementia, nerve problems, cracking sores at the corners of the mouth, and impaired immune system. Can also lead to malabsorption making the deficiency worse.	Folic acid supplementations increase the body's requirements for B12. Large dose of B6 increase requirements for folic acid. Digestive enzymes can bind with folic acid making it harder to absorb.	Leafy green vegetables, legumes, citrus fruits, beets, whole grains.	Folic acid supplementation plays a crucial role in preventing neural tube defects in pregnancy
B12	Involved in the nervous system and immune system, helps with DNA synthesis and red blood cell formation.	Deficiency symptoms include macrocytic anemia, memory loss, depression, confusion, delirium, swelling of the tongue, changes in skin colour, permanent neurological damage if left too long, impaired ability to fight bacterial infections	Folic acid given without B12 can aggravate a B12 deficiency and mask the blood test results for determining B12 deficiency.	Meat, fish, poultry, dairy, eggs.	It typically takes 3-5 years to completely exhaust B12 stores. B12 is made in the intestines by bacteria. As we age our ability to make B12 is greatly reduced. (Intramuscular shots are the best way to treat

Vitamins

	What it does in the body	Symptoms of deficiency	Interactions with other nutrients	Foods high in nutrient	Interesting Facts
Fat Soluble Vitamins					
Vitamin A	Vitamin A is needed for the pigment in your eyes that allow you to see.	Signs of vitamin A deficiency include night blindness, loss of appetite, slow growth, bumpy red rash on the backs of upper arms, problems with sperm production, poor immune function, increased susceptibility to infection, and more serious eye conditions including blindness.	Vitamin E enhances intestinal absorption of vitamin A so that lower doses can be taken. Zinc helps transport Vitamin A around the body so zinc deficiency decreases blood levels of Vitamin A.	Fish oils, dairy products, eggs, and vitamin A fortified foods.	Carrots are good for your eyes. They contain a compound, called beta carotene, that can be converted to Vitamin A in your body.
Vitamin D	Vitamin D acts as a precursor to hormones, increases absorption of calcium and phosphorous in the gut, promotes strong bones, helps regulate insulin, helps immune system regulation and disease prevention including cancer, MS, psoriasis, and osteoporosis.	Severe deficiency in children is called rickets – soft deformed bones, muscle weakness, and dental problems. In adults it is called osteomalacia – soft bones, bone pain, muscle weakness, chronic low back pain, fatigue, and head sweating.	Calcium: vitamin D increases its absorption increasing the risk of having high calcium in the blood or urine	Oily fish – mackerel, salmon, and sardines, and vitamin D fortified foods (milk, orange juice, cereals and bread)	Deficiency symptoms can appear like fibromyalgia, depression, and chronic fatigue syndrome. Deficiency is common in northern climates as the body can synthesize vitamin D from sunlight.

Vitamins

	What it does in the body	Symptoms of deficiency	Interactions with other nutrients	Foods high in nutrient	Interesting Facts
Fat Soluble Vitamins					
Vitamin E	Vitamin E is a strong antioxidant, helps to stabilize the outer layer of the cell; it prevents blood clotting and has anti-inflammatory effects. At moderate doses it can enhance immune function.	Severe deficiency can lead to neuromuscular problems, and damage to the retina of the eye. It is rare to be severely deficient unless a person has a fat absorption problem, however, less than optimal levels could contribute to a wide range of conditions.	Large doses of E could compromise Vitamin K status. Vitamin E & C work together and taking one increases the requirements of the other. Iron prevents proper absorption of E.	Nuts, seeds, unprocessed vegetable oils (wheat germ oil, almond oil, and sunflower oil), whole grains, egg yolks, and leafy green vegetables.	If you are eating a lot of deep fried foods, you are not getting much Vitamin E. Vitamin E is destroyed by frying.
Vitamin K	Vitamin K helps with blood clotting and bone building.	Severe deficiency of vitamin K can lead to severe bleeding episodes, while being somewhat low in vitamin K may lead to bone loss or osteoporosis and calcium build up in the arteries	Too much vitamin E could put someone who is low in vitamin K at risk for bleeding. Too much vitamin A can interfere with vitamin K.	Leafy green vegetables (main source), natto (fermented soy), cheese, butter, eggs, meat	There are two natural forms of Vitamin K. One (phylloquinone) can be produced in the intestines. Cultured milk products, like yogurt can increase its production.

Minerals

	What it does in the body	Symptoms of deficiency	Interactions with other nutrients	Foods high in nutrient	Interesting Facts
Calcium	Strengthens bones and teeth, needed for muscle contraction, and breaking down stored sugars from the liver and muscles	Long term low calcium intake results in bone loss (osteoporosis) and in children rickets occasionally (but more from vitamin D deficiency)	Some research has shown that taking high levels of calcium increases the requirement for magnesium. High calcium doses might interfere with iron absorption and should be taken apart.	Dairy products, canned sardines or salmon with bones, kale, broccoli, collard greens, mustard greens, turnip greens, bok-choy, sesame seeds, black strap molasses, calcium fortified foods	Foods that are high in calcium but also high in oxalates (naturally occurring organic acids) like spinach aren't a good source of calcium because the oxalates prevent the calcium from being absorbed.
Iron	Iron plays an important role in making energy for the body. It's also found in red blood cells and muscle cells where it helps to transport oxygen. Iron also helps with the making of protein, hormones, neurotransmitters, and collagen	Symptoms of deficiency can include: anemia, fatigue, weakness, headaches, apathy, pallor, sensitivity to cold, pale skin, unmotivated and apathetic, trouble paying attention, an appetite for ice, clay, dirt, paste or other non-food substances	Vitamin C enhances iron absorption. Oxalates in foods inhibit the absorption of iron.	Most absorbed from meats, fish and poultry, eggs and grains have some iron and dark greens and some fruit have iron.	Iron supplements can be constipating, so remember to drink lots of water and do not be alarmed if you have darker stools, it is a common effect.

Minerals

	What it does in the body	Symptoms of deficiency	Interactions with other nutrients	Foods high in nutrient	Interesting Facts
Magnesium	Magnesium is needed for over 300 enzymes in the body, It's needed to make energy, and it's needed to make your heart and nerves work. It helps to relax muscles and make blood vessels bigger. It is also involved in the breakdown of fats and sugars in the body.	Mild-Moderate magnesium deficiency symptoms: anxiety, depression, fatigue, insomnia, irritability, panic attacks, muscle cramps and twitches, headaches, chest tightness, difficulty concentrating, palpitations, memory loss, etc. Severe deficiency: muscle weakness, vertigo, seizures, hallucinations, stupor, and coma.	Calcium: with large amounts of calcium supplementation it may increase the magnesium requirements of the body. Magnesium and B6 work together to increase each other's uptake. Magnesium is required to turn B1 into its active form. Large doses of zinc can decrease magnesium absorption.	Nuts, whole grains, legumes, green leafy vegetables, fish, meat, and dairy products	More than 80% of magnesium is lost in refining whole-wheat flour to white flour, and 50-70% of the magnesium is lost in vegetable cooking water. Some people are chronically depleted in magnesium. In the body, magnesium is found inside the cell however it is easily pushed out of the cell by lead, mercury and arsenic.
Chloride	Chloride is an electrolyte like sodium and potassium and it helps maintain fluid balance in the body. In the stomach chloride is part of hydrochloric acid, which is needed for protein digestion.	You can lose a lot of chloride from heavy sweating, and chronic diarrhea and vomiting.	Chloride is a member of the halide family in chemistry which displaces another halide, iodine, in the body hindering its usage and absorption.	Salt, soy sauce, meat, milk, eggs, lots in processed foods	We are overexposed to chloride (in the form of chlorine) in our drinking water.

Minerals

	What it does in the body	Symptoms of deficiency	Interactions with other nutrients	Foods high in nutrient	Interesting Facts
Sodium	Helps nerves function and muscle contraction. Plays a large role in fluid regulation and hydration of the body.	Sodium can be lost to heavy sweating, chronic diarrhea, and vomiting. Symptoms of deficiency include muscle cramps, mental apathy, and loss of appetite.	Potassium: High potassium intake increases sodium output in the urine.	Salt, soy sauce, meat, milk, eggs, lots in processed foods	Replacing electrolytes after doing physical labor in hot conditions should include potassium and sodium chloride (salt). Too much sodium is a cause of hypertension.
Zinc	Zinc is a cofactor to many enzymes and is involved in many reactions in the body including DNA and protein synthesis. Zinc is needed for growing, vision, hearing, taste, to make sperm, sexual development, immune function and wound healing. Zinc is also a good antioxidant, anti-inflammatory, and anti-viral.	Signs of deficiency can include impaired taste, anorexia, pica (eating of non-foods like dirt), depression, jitteriness, impaired mental concentration, short stature, skin problems, diarrhea, erectile dysfunction, night blindness, low sperm count, low testosterone, anemia, poor wound healing, light sensitivity, increased susceptibility to infections, hair loss	Large to moderate doses of zinc for a prolonged period can cause copper deficiency. Zinc and Iron can compete to be absorbed so it is advisable to take them at separate times. Zinc is needed to transport vitamin A, therefore zinc might be needed to raise vitamin A.	Seafood, meats, whole grains, wheat germ, wheat bran, dairy, legumes, peanuts, egg yolk, nuts and seeds.	Signs of mild zinc deficiencies can be seen on your nails, ever wonder what those white spots are?

104

Minerals

	What it does in the body	Symptoms of deficiency	Interactions with other nutrients	Foods high in nutrient	Interesting Facts
Copper	Copper helps strengthen connective tissue, promotes wound healing, and plays a role in the immune system, the pumping of the heart; bone building, making skin pigment, and regulating cholesterol and blood sugar levels.	Deficiency symptoms include: slowed growth, anemia, bone problems like osteoporosis, and decreased resistance against infections, and blood sugar problems.	Zinc interferes with copper absorption. Iron competes with copper for absorption. Alpha lipoic acid increases excretion of copper in the urine. Molybdenum binds with copper and then it can't be absorbed.	Fish, meat, poultry, eggs, nuts, legumes, whole grains, vegetables and fruit.	Copper can leach into food and drinking water through copper pipes and cookware, careful not to have excessive amounts. Pressure treated wood is a large source of copper exposure.
Selenium	Selenium is a cofactor of gluathione, a major antioxidant in the body. Selenium is good for the immune system and has antiviral properties; it also plays a role in thyroid hormone function.	Selenium deficiency is related to Keshan disease, a heart disease that affected many children in China. Other deficiency symptoms include a weakened heart, muscle pain and weakness, white fingernail beds, and elevated liver enzymes.	Giving selenium to people with low iodine can trigger hypothyroidism. Taking large amounts of essential fatty acids like fish oils increases the requirement for selenium.	Meat, fish, whole grains, legumes, brazil nuts, garlic, mushrooms and asparagus.	Whole wheat contains 5 times more selenium than refined flour.
Chromium	Chromium is needed to help insulin do its job of regulating blood sugar. Chromium also has an effect on the brain chemical serotonin.	Deficiency symptoms include blood sugar problems, weight loss, nerve pain in the lower legs, and confusion.		Whole grains and eggs	40-70% of chromium is lost when whole wheat is refined to white flour.

Minerals

	What it does in the body	Symptoms of deficiency	Interactions with other nutrients	Foods high in nutrient	Interesting Facts
Potassium	Potassium is needed to make your nerves, heart, muscles work, and it plays a role in blood pressure also. It is one of the electrolytes that is necessary to keep you properly hydrated.	Deficiency symptoms include fatigue, weakness, muscle cramps, palpitations, irregular heartbeats, high blood pressure and dizziness from lying to standing up.	Magnesium is essential to get potassium into our cells and so low potassium won't be helped by supplementation without magnesium also (if you are low in magnesium). Higher potassium intake can help you urinate more sodium, which is protective from the blood pressure raising effects of sodium.	Fruits and vegetables: bananas, oranges, grapefruit, pineapple, apples, apricots, squash, avocados, spinach and sweet potatoes, beans, whole grains, milk, fish, meat, and black strap molasses.	50% of the potassium can be lost in the water when foods are boiled.
Iodine	Iodine is an important component of thyroid hormones.	Iodine deficiency during pregnancy cause irreversible brain damage in infants. With chronic iodine deficiency people can develop goiter, hypothyroidism, poor hearing, and reduced intelligence.	High intake of non-iodized salt could deplete iodine. Chlorine and bromine can often interact and reduce iodine available for proper thyroid function.	Milk, cheese, meat, fish, poultry, eggs, kelp and other seaweeds, and iodized salt.	The large amounts of iodine in milk products are from the iodine based sanitizing solutions used on the cow's udders and for the milking equipment. The Great Lakes Region is called the "Goiter Belt" due to a deficiency of iodine in the soil.

Numerous people are deficient in nutrients. The greatest cause has not been from lack of exposure but actually from sensitivity to the mineral. These sensitivities can result in poor absorption, decreased energy, poor memory, headaches and multiple allergies. The Elimination Allergy Technique is an effective treatment for removing sensitivities (*please refer to EAT for more information*). Multi-mineral sensitivity can also occur from excess exposure to certain minerals (magnesium, zinc, selenium etc.) and mineral deficiencies from heavy metal accumulation (*please refer to Heavy Metals for more information*).

References:
1. Gaby, AR. Nutritional Medicine. Concord, NH: Fritz Perlberg Publishing, 2011.
2. Haas, E.M. "Staying Healthy With Nutrition: The Complete Guide to Diet and Nutritional Medicine." (2006)
3. Whitney, EN, CB Cataldo, and SR Rolfes. Understanding Normal and Clinical Nutrition. 6th ed., Belmont, CA: Wadsworth/Thomson Learning, 2002.

Hygiene

A dirty history

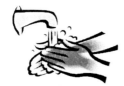

According to the Center of Disease Control, washing one's hands on a regular basis is the most effective and overlooked way to prevent infection. It was not until 1847, when the observations which lead to the practice of hand washing in medical clinics were made by Dr. Semmelweis. While working at an obstetrics clinic, Dr. Semmelweis was alarmed by the amount of mothers suffering from fatal childbed fever following delivery. The incidence was significantly higher in births assisted by medical students than by midwives. Dr. Semmelweis discovered that medical students helping with childbirth did so after performing autopsies on patients who died from sepsis. Armed with this knowledge, mortality rates dropped by 20-fold in 3 months, after a strict hand-washing policy with a chlorinated antiseptic solution was instituted. We have, of course, come a long way since 1847 and yet improper hand washing continues to significantly contribute to disease transmission.

The mouth is a major gateway for microorganisms to enter the bloodstream. Routine practices of washing hands with soap for at least 15 seconds, prior to consuming or preparing food can decrease the entrance of disease causing bacteria and germs into the body. Cleaning your hands after you use the bathroom or changing a diaper are all part of preventative methods. Covering your mouth and nose when you sneeze or cough can help stop the spread of germ-filled droplets into the air. Avoid touching your eyes and nose as microorganisms can enter the body through these sites. Colds and flu are often transmitted this way. The Hand, Foot and Mouth disease virus is spread when infected persons touch objects and surfaces that are then touched by others. Taking hygienic precautions is important not only to protect yourself but also to prevent infection of those around you. Mary Mallon was responsible for several outbreaks of typhoid fever in the United States in the early 1900s. She was identified as an asymptomatic carrier of the pathogen and presumed to have infected over 53 people during her career as a cook. Infamous Typhoid Mary's personal contact with food and those around her is a prime example of the necessity to practice preventative methods.

Hand washing is only the first step in proper personal hygiene. Bathing regularly and wearing clean clothes keeps your body free of dirt, germs and lice. Wearing shower shoes in public facilities can decrease the spread of fungal infections. Properly airing out your shower shoes and allowing them to dry ensures that mold and fungus do not grow in your protective gear. Parasitic and fungal infections can also be found on clothes. Washing clothes regularly is important to keep the skin clean and prevent microbial accumulation on the material. Washing machines are great for cleaning clothing but they can also be a source of germs. Keeping the lid open after a wash allows for proper drying of the machine and restricts any growth of mold and fungi from standing water in the machine. Running an empty wash cycle with soap and hot water once a month, helps keep the machine free of bacteria and spores. (Please note: continuous washing of undergarments in only cold water can contribute to chronic yeast infections and urinary tract infections. Do not be afraid to add some hot water on a routine basis). Hockey and football equipment, shower shoes and washing machines, create the perfect wet environment to harbor growth. Do you ever wonder where that smell is from? Airing out the equipment and spraying it with white vinegar should be practiced after each use!

Regular grooming methods of hair and nails can help prevent dirt accumulation and infestation of infectious agents. The buildup of oils on the face from the skin and hair can lead to acne break-outs especially around the hairline. Cleaning and brushing teeth daily is an excellent habit to prevent bad breath and keep gums healthy. Food particles that remain in the mouth form a medium for germs to grow and cause gingivitis, dental caries and periodontal disease. Proper oral hygiene can often be overlooked. One of the problems associated with gum disease is an increased risk for heart complications. Dental procedures with increased bleeding from gum disease can allow bacteria to enter the bloodstream and cause infection in other parts of the body, specifically to heart valves. This outcome can be avoided, by proper teeth care.

Domestic hygiene is paramount to avoiding disease. Keep living areas clean and free from dirt, flies and germs help prevent the spread of illness. Cooking utensils, pots, plates and cups should be kept clean as mold can grow on leftover food. Food and water can be a major source of contamination leading to illness. Use clean water sources for drinking, cooking, bathing and washing (preferably filtered). Wash fruits and vegetables before consumption with a light soap to remove pesticides and microorganisms. Fresh fruits and vegetables can be contaminated if they are washed or irrigated with dirty water. During food processing microbes can be introduced by a person with an infection, like Typhoid Mary, or by cross contamination from raw products. *Shigella* bacteria, *hepatitis* A virus and *norovirus* can be caused by the unwashed hands of food handlers who are themselves infected. Using the same knife, cutting board or utensils without washing, can transfer microorganisms from one food to another. Cooked food can be re-contaminated if it comes in contact with raw food or raw food drippings. Food left out overnight can be highly infectious the next day;

refrigeration or freezing prevents bacteria growth. Properly heating food to 160°F or 78°C can kill parasites, viruses and bacteria (Please note: in pregnancy food must always be cooked well-done prior to consumption). Safe and proper methods are important when handling and preparing food.

Many diseases and conditions can be prevented or controlled through appropriate practice of high standards of personal and domestic hygiene.

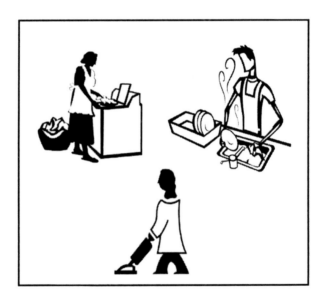

References:
1. Centers for Disease Control and Prevention: www.cdc.gov
2. http://infectiousdiseases.about.com/od/prevention/a/history_hygiene.htm
3. http://history1900s.about.com/od/1900s/a/typhoidmary.htm

Exercise

A love hate relationship

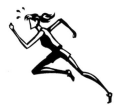
We all know that exercise is encouraged as a natural means of disease prevention. The World Health Organization has identified physical inactivity as the fourth leading risk factor for global mortality (behind high blood pressure, tobacco use and high blood glucose). Half of the body's functional decline observed between the ages of 30 and 70 is due to an inactive lifestyle and not to aging itself.

Physical activity can help prevent chronic disease including Type II diabetes, obesity, cancer and cardiovascular disease. Regular exercise strengthens your heart muscle, lowers blood pressure, enhances blood flow, reduces your resting heart rate, increases high-density lipoproteins (HDL, good cholesterol) and lowers low-density lipoproteins (LDL, bad cholesterol). All of these benefits reduce the risk of stroke, heart disease and hypertension.

Exercise can help improve self-esteem, energy, stress and resilience to stress. During physical activity, the body releases chemicals called endorphins that can directly elevate your mood. The feelings that follow a workout are often described as "euphoric" and are accompanied by an energizing outlook. Incorporating physical activity into your schedule routinely helps you feel better about yourself and promotes a positive cycle. Exercise helps the body to use calories more efficiently, increases basal metabolic rate, reduces appetite and body fat, all aiding with weight loss and weight control.

Physical activity is essential for healthy growth and development. It is never too early to encourage healthy habits. In childhood, regular physical activity improves development of cardiovascular fitness, strength and bone density. In adulthood, weight-bearing physical activity reduces the rate of bone loss associated with osteoporosis. Regular exercise maintains strength and flexibility, balance and coordination and helps reduce the risk of falls with age. Physical activity prolongs good health and independence.

Finding the time in your daily schedule to exercise can often be difficult. There are 1440 minutes in one day. According to the revised Canadian Physical Activity Guidelines released by the CSEP (the Canadian Society for Exercise Physiology) children (ages 5 to 11) and youth (ages 12 to 17) are recommended to:

- accumulate at least 60 minutes of moderate to vigorous intensity physical activity daily
- include vigorous-intensity activities at least 3 days per week.

111

- include activities that strengthen muscle and bone at least 3 days per week.

Adults aged 18 to 64 should accumulate at least 150 minutes of moderate to vigorous aerobic physical activity per week, in 10 minutes bouts or more. This can include a brisk walk, jogging, cycling and dancing. Stretching and weight training strengthens your body and improves your fitness level.

Regular physical activity helps protect you against some of the leading causes of illness and should be incorporated into a healthy lifestyle. To develop a new habit it takes 21 days, so work up to the new regulations. Start slow and increase the length of time and intensity. After 21 days reassess your weight, your energy, your blood pressure and think about how you feel (*please refer to Changing Habits*).

References:
1. Public Health Agency of Canada: http://www.phac-aspc.gc.ca/hp-ps/hl-mvs/pa-ap/index-eng.php
2. World Health Organization: http://www.who.int/dietphysicalactivity/pa/en/index.html
3. http://www.cbc.ca/news/health/story/2011/01/24/fitness-guidelines.html

Prescription Drugs

Things to Consider

The use and abuse of drugs is prevalent throughout history. Natural product extracts from botanical plants provided the main source of medicines in the early centuries. In the later part of the nineteenth century, biologically active organic molecules were isolated from plants. For example, salicylic acid, the precursor of aspirin was isolated in 1874 from willow bark. Potent painkillers, morphine and codeine, were isolated from the opium poppy. The leaves of purple foxglove provided digitalis for heart disease. The active ingredients that were found in plants are now synthesized on a massive scale to produce pharmaceutical drugs.

Next to oil companies and the war industry, pharmaceutical companies are the most profitable industry in the world: $643 billion worldwide were spent on drugs in 2006. Pharmaceutical companies focus on producing artificial substances that can be patented. Little interest is given to researching natural substances because they cannot be patented. In order to manufacture or patent their own product, an additional molecule is often attached to the synthesized active ingredient (a copy of the active ingredient found in the natural substance). This new substance may look similar to the natural form however it does not entirely act the same. The synthetic molecule with the foreign side chain affects how it is metabolized in the body and how it acts (*please refer to Hormones for more information*).

With all the money spent on research in the pharmaceutical industry we often believe that prescription drugs should be exceptionally safe. That however, is not the case. Not only do pharmaceutical drugs tend to have multiple side effects, but they are also unpredictable when mixed with each other. Many 'adverse events' can occur from medication being improperly administered. It is estimated that over one million people are injured and **285,000 die** from the injuries sustained while hospitalized in the US in one year. A substantial percentage of those are caused by medication mishaps. In a 2004 Canadian study, they found **185,000 incidences** of adverse events in hospitals. These events were more likely to happen in older patients who coincidentally tend to be on more medications. In the US the total number of drug related deaths now surpasses fatalities from car accidents. Interestingly, in 2011 an article published in the Journal of Medical Ethics revealed a disturbing trend in the amount of retractions from previously published journal articles. Retractions can occur because of errors in data, collection of statistics or fraud. From 2001 to 2006 there was a 500 percent increase in the amount of retractions. Based on recent patterns, a minimum of 360 articles was predicted to be retracted in 2011. The number of retractions brings forth many ethical concerns regarding faulty research. It also begs the question of whether the evidence for the safety of certain pharmaceutical drugs is truly legitimate. **Prescription drug errors are actually considered the leading cause of death.** A 2003 report revealed that 783,936 deaths are the result of medication in the US alone and over 2 million worldwide every year.

Prescription drug addiction is a growing problem. Since the medications were originally ordered by a doctor, prescription drug abuse is seen differently than street drug abuse. Prescription drugs can also lead to addiction. Prescription medications such as pain relievers, tranquilizers, stimulants and sedatives become addicting in the same way street drugs do. The medication changes the brain's chemistry, making it less effective at producing chemicals like dopamine or endorphins, the pleasure neurotransmitters. Since the brain has stopped producing these chemicals itself, they must be introduced through another source. At this point, the prescription drug addict has become physically dependent on the medication. A person addicted to prescription drugs may experience anxiety, depression and difficulty sleeping or sleeping too much, loss of interest in relationships with friends or family members, or withdrawal symptoms when they try to stop using the medication on their own. These may be the symptoms they originally began taking the medication for.

Top Ten Abused Prescription Drugs

- Ambien (zolpidem) ~Insomnia
- Seroquel (quetiapine) ~Antipsychotic
- Dilaudid (hydromorphone) ~Pain
- Xanax (alprazolam) ~Antianxiety
- Desoyxn (methamphetamine) ~Stimulant
- Narcotic syrups (codeine and hydrocodone)~Neurological Suppressant
- Adderall (mixed amphetamine salts) ~Stimulant
- Laudanum (opium tincture) ~Pain
- OxyContin (oxycodone) ~Pain
- Opana (oxymorphone) ~Pain

Pharmaceuticals can have significant toxic effects to the body. Unexpected side effects, or interactions, with other medications can often occur. In many cases, these medications can inhibit the function of the body's natural detoxification pathways leading to excess amounts remaining in your system for longer periods of time. The impact your medications can have on your health should not be easily dismissed. Your ND, as part of their training, has been educated on drug to drug interactions and drug to herb interactions. All research on drugs is held to the highest standard of investigation which is the double blind studies, however once more than 2 prescription medications have been prescribed the outcome is mostly unknown.

Prescription drug trends have increased exponentially over the past 20 years. In 2011 the total expenditure in Canada is forecasted at $32 billion dollars. Non-

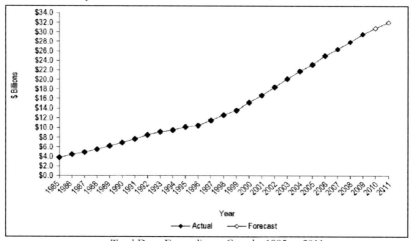

Total Drug Expenditure, Canada, 1985 to 2011
https://secure.cihi.ca/free_products/DEIC_1985_2011_EN.pdf

prescribed drugs (i.e. over the counter medications, supplements etc.) only accounted for 16% of the total. From 1985 to 2009, prescribed drug expenditure grew from $2.6 billion to $24.8 billion while non-prescribed drugs increased from $1.2 billion to $4.8 billion. Accounting for a small portion of drug trends in Canada.

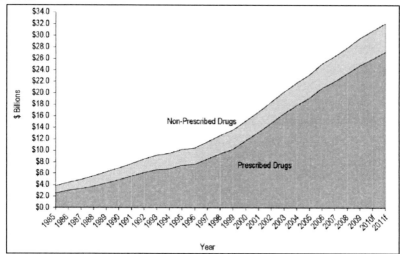

Total Drug Expenditure, by Type (Prescribed and Non-Prescribed), Canada, 1985 to 2011
https://secure.cihi.ca/free_products/DEIC_1985_2011_EN.pdf

Canadians use more prescriptions than ever before. According to Statistics Canada in 2005, pharmacists dispensed on average 35 prescriptions per person aged 60 to 79 and 74 prescriptions for patients aged 80 or older. Currently, there is an overall average of **14 prescriptions per Canadian** citizen. This data stresses the need to be concerned about your health and to begin long-term maintenance at an early age. Waiting until your health declines can ultimately lead to astronomical costs to you and your family.

With the substantial growth in prescription drug use, the real and hidden truth behind publication bias should be exposed. The practice of selectively publishing the results of trials that beneficially serve an agenda is a systematic flaw in medicine. The bias ultimately includes positive results and not negative ones, the lack of retractions from fraudulent studies and the influences of funding. A shocking half of all completed trials on medical treatments currently prescribed have never been published. Positive results are two times more likely to be found in the literature. This publication prejudice is quite serious as the end result is death if choices are continuously being made with inaccurate information and recommendations.

In 1980, a study conducted on a heart arrhythmia drug called lorcainade had quite negative results. Of the 100 participants, 50% received the drug. Among the treatment group 10 died in comparison to the one death from the placebo group. The commercialization of the drug was abandoned although the trial was never published. Similar arrhythmic drugs were created and marketed over the next 10 years by other competitive pharmaceutical companies. An estimated 100,000 deaths occurred in the U.S. alone before the drugs were found as the cause. This is merely one example of the price of publication bias as the negative results from the lorcainade trial may have provided an early warning if they had been available.

The flu drug, Tamiflu, is currently anticipated as the main treatment for a flu pandemic. Remarkably the science behind Tamiflu is not available. Of the 10 studies conducted, **eight** have never been released. In 2012, Cochrane (an organization well known for their scientific reviews) attempted to update their data on influenza management. The previous assessment of Tamiflu was from 2009. Despite best efforts, the group was unable to get the manufacturer (Roche) to release the missing 8 clinical trials of Tamiflu. In collaboration with the British Medical Journal (BMJ), Cochrane revealed this issue to the public. The BMJ Open Data Campaign site contains links with Cochrane's communications with Roche, the CDC and the WHO, all of which suggests their awareness and continued support of Tamiflu, regardless of full scientific disclosure.

The publication bias is a definite flaw. All research is not published and negative results from pharmaceutically funded trials will rarely be seen. With the amount

116

of data missing and unavailable there certainly cannot be a claim or guarantee of a drug's safety and effectiveness. Knowledge is power, be aware of the ill effects and addicting possibilities of prescription medications.

The following video link is a humorous depiction of a pharmaceutical drug. Refer to http://www.youtube.com/watch?v=yLR2OKesTw0 or Google Progenitorivox.

References:
1. http://uga-cdd.org/background.php
2. http://www.thegooddrugsguide.com/addiction-types/drug-addiction/prescription-drug-abuse.htm
3. http://psychcentral.com/blog/archives/2011/08/10/retractions-of-scientific-research-papers-going-up/
4. http://www.whale.to/a/dean.html
5. http://www.statcan.gc.ca/pub/82-003-x/2009001/article/10801/findings-resultats-eng.htm
6. https://secure.cihi.ca/free_products/DEIC_1985_2011_EN.pdf
7. Ben Goldacre: What doctors don't know about the drugs they prescribe. Sept 27, 2012. Ted Talks Director. http://www.youtube.com/watch?v=RKmxL8VYy0M
8. Mercola. Publication Bias-the Hidden Systematic Flaw in Medicine that Can Threaten Your Life. February 13, 2013. http://articles.mercola.com/sites/articles/archive/2013/02/13/publication-bias.aspx

Water Quantity

Are you drying up?

 Our bodies are primarily dependent on water to function. Water makes up 60% of our body weight. Every system in our body uses water to carry nutrients to our cells and to remove toxins.

Water is an essential part of our bodies' natural detoxification processes. Water is lost through perspiration, respiration, urination and digestion. Inadequate amounts can lead to dehydration that prevents proper daily function and can cause decreased energy, light headedness, dry mouth, heart palpitations, nausea and vomiting. If left untreated, severe dehydration can result in seizures, brain damage and even death. It is very important to replenish your water supply to prevent these negative complications. Interestingly, one milliliter of water is needed to metabolize one calorie from the food we eat. Hunger and thirst can often send similar neurological signals to the brain and so occasionally we are actually thirsty at times when we feel hungry. Try a glass of water and see if it helps satisfy your craving.

How do we know how much water we are losing per day? The average person will lose about 1 liter (approximately 4 cups) through sweating, breathing and bowel movements and about 1.5 liters (roughly 6 cups) from urinary output. Food can usually account for about 20% of fluid intake. If you consume about 2 liters of water daily (nearly 8 cups), you can sufficiently replace the amount of water lost through elimination pathways. Exercise increases perspiration, so an extra 2 cups may be required depending on the intensity of the activity to compensate for the extra fluid loss. Hot environments also lead to increased sweating. Illness, accompanied by fever, vomiting, diarrhea or urinary tract infections will lead to additional fluids loss from the body. Your intake must be increased in these situations.

It is possible to drink too much water. The kidneys play an important role in water excretion. When the kidneys fail to remove the excess water, the mineral content in our blood becomes diluted. This can result in low sodium levels, a condition called hyponatremia. Endurance athletes and marathon runners are more at risk for this. Sodium is just one example of an electrolyte used by the body. Electrolytes are essential chemical substances necessary for all cells. Maintaining a proper balance is vital for daily function especially during the summer. The elderly are in particular more susceptible to humid temperatures. In general, excessive thirst and increased urination can be indications of a more serious condition.

References:

1. MayoClinic: http://www.mayoclinic.com/health/water/NU00283
2. Canadian Living : http://www.canadianliving.com/health/nutrition/water_how_much_should_you_drink_every_day.php
3. http://www.livestrong.com/article/41036-replace-electrolytes/#ixzz1tF6Jfa8k

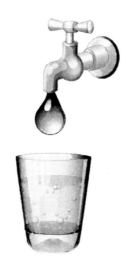

Obesity and Body Mass Index

Stats, Stats and more Stats

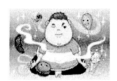 According to Statistics Canada, two out of every three adults are either overweight or obese. Poor eating habits and physical inactivity are critical concerns to public health. In the U.S., two-thirds of the population is obese. A new study from the Centers for Disease Control and Prevention (CDC) on obesity data from 2007 to 2009, found an estimated 34 percent of Americans are obese compared to 24 percent of Canadians. Interestingly Pacific Island Nations, including Samoa, have the worst obesity problem in the world. Since the average Samoan male is considered to be obese, Samoa Air now asks passengers to declare their personal weight during booking. They are the world's first carrier to charge passengers by their weight rather than per seat. This may be the progressing concept of the future.

Unfortunately, adults are not the only ones plagued by this epidemic. Approximately 17% (or 12.5 million) of children and adolescents aged 2-19 years are obese in the U.S and 8.6% of children and youth aged 6-17 are obese in Canada. Obesity rates in children and youth have tripled over the last 25 years in Canada. Teenagers who are obese have an 80% chance of remaining overweight or obese as adults. Weight problems in childhood are likely to persist into adult years. The prevalence of this disease and the associated health consequences are alarming.

Overweight and obesity ranges are determined by using weight and height to calculate the "body mass index" (BMI). This number correlates with the amount of body fat a person may have. An adult who has a BMI between 25 and 29.9 is considered overweight while an adult with a BMI of 30 or higher is considered obese. As weight increases, the risks for developing multiple disease conditions also increase. These can include coronary heart disease, stroke, type II diabetes, hypertension, dyslipidemia, sleep apnea, respiratory problems, osteoarthritis, liver and gallbladder disease, infertility and some cancers including endometrial, breast and colon. Excessive weight can also impact emotional and social health; low self-esteem, negative body image and depression.

Waist Circumference (WC) is another indicator associated with health risk. Excess fat deposited around the waist and upper body has been linked with a greater risk of disease compared to fat around the hip and thigh areas. For example, a WC of 102 cm or more in men and 88 cm or more for women have a higher risk of developing high blood pressure, diabetes and heart disease. Your risk of developing health problems increases as BMI and WC measurements increase.

Several factors have contributed to the increase in the number of overweight and obese individuals within the population. Changes in work, society and leisure to name a few, have affected eating patterns and physical activity. The greater availability of high-caloric dense food, sugar drinks, larger portion sizes and inexpensive prices have each played a role. The increased use of automated transport, less physically demanding work and the development of more passive leisure activities have had effects on weight statistics. Fewer children and youth are walking to and from school as a result of safety concerns today.

Watching TV or playing video games has been found to have a direct correlation with weight gain. Entertainment increases caloric consumption and influences food choices. One eats more and faster when excited, engaged or stressed by a program. Eating for pleasure and comfort instead of necessity is very much the norm. The current perception of food has inadvertently created challenges for maintaining a healthy weight.

Obesity is one of the leading factors contributing to increased risk of developing serious health problems.

References:
1. Centers for Disease Control and Prevention: http://www.cdc.gov/obesity/childhood/problem.html
2. Health Canada: http://www.healthycanadians.gc.ca/init/kids-enfants/obesit/index-eng.php
3. http://www.hc-sc.gc.ca/hl-vs/iyh-vsv/life-vie/obes-eng.php
4. http://www.cdc.gov/obesity/data/trends.html
5. http://www.phac-aspc.gc.ca/hp-ps/hl-mvs/oic-oac/index-eng.php
6. http://www.huffingtonpost.com/2011/03/02/us-obesity-rate-much-high_n_830272.html
7. Ogden, C. L., Carroll, M. D., Kit, B.K., & Flegal, K. M. (2012). Prevalence of obesity and trends in body mass index among U.S. children and adolescents, 1999-2010. Journal of the American Medical Association, 307(5), 483-490.
8. http://www.newsmax.com/Health-News/airline-overweight-passengers-charges/2013/04/03/id/497665
9. http://www.economist.com/blogs/gulliver/2013/04/heavy-passengers

Chapter 5

Disease Causing Factors: Body

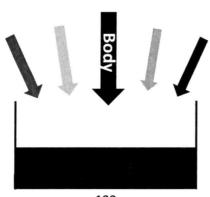

Circulation and Blood Pressure

The most used muscle

The circulatory system is vital to the proper function of the human body. Our blood plays an important role in maintaining homeostasis (balance) by bringing essential nutrients and oxygen to our organs and many parts of the body. With poor circulation, beneficial oxygen and healthy nutrients do not reach necessary areas of the body. While harmful metabolic substances, like carbon monoxide and dioxide, become entrapped in tissues leading to disease.

Excess fat and cholesterol can build up on the walls of arteries, forming a substance known as plaque. Plaque narrows arteries and reduces blood flow. If left untreated, blocked blood flow can cause tissue death. Legs are often affected by decreased circulation leading to symptoms of claudication, a dull cramping pain in the calf muscle that comes on after walking long distances and is relieved by rest. As the condition worsens, the distance becomes shorter and shorter. Other signs of decreased circulation can include: numbness or tingling in the feet and toes, changes in skin colour or temperature, skin damage, or infections that do not heal as well as they should.

Lack of physical activity, smoking, high blood pressure and obesity are all risk factors known for contributing to poor circulation. Other less known factors found to narrow arteries and increase plaque formation include heavy metals, infection, inflammation, hypercoagulability (sticky blood), nitric oxide deficiency and oxalate crystal formation (stone formation) [*please refer to Heart Disease for more specific information on these causes*]. These factors are also associated with common diseases observed with problems in circulation, for example, diabetes, varicose veins, venous thrombosis, pregnancy, atherosclerosis, edema, high or low blood pressure and multiple sclerosis. Improper nutrition, increased acidic toxins and changes in pH (acid/base balance in the body) are also believed to play a role in circulation. In the environment, we are exposed to free radicals that are known to damage cells. Our oxygen supply and our diet, especially the consumption of soft drinks, are potential sources of free radicals. Proper food consumption of vitamins, minerals, amino acids and essential fatty acids are important to decrease acidity in the body, neutralize free radicals, strengthen the integrity of our cells and prevent break down in veins, arteries and capillaries.

Traditionally in Chinese Medicine, the major activity of blood is to circulate continuously through the body, nourishing, maintaining and moistening. When either the entire body or a particular organ is insufficiently nourished, a deficiency can result leading to signs of paleness, lusterless face, dizziness and dry skin.

123

However, when blood becomes obstructed, this form of stagnant blood can cause sharp, stabbing pains. Understanding the importance of blood to the function of the body allows us to see how low energy, irregular heartbeats, shortness of breath, lack of stamina and sluggish memory can be indications of blood failing to nourish and maintain the body.

The concerns of poor circulation are often believed to begin in adulthood. Unfortunately, this is not the case. Dr. Sanaz Piran, an internal medicine resident at McMaster University in Hamilton, Ontario, has reported early onset of atherosclerosis in children too. As obesity, lack of physical activity and improper diet are also growing problems in the young population. These risk factors may allow for children to be more susceptible for developing circulatory problems. The article reviewed data on 3,620 children aged 5 to 18 and found early signs of atherosclerosis in the children. A measurement of the amount of plaque on artery walls by ultrasound, known as CIMT (Carotid artery intima media thickness), is used as a marker for atherosclerosis and heart disease in adults. In 2010, another study of 6-19 year old obese children, found CIMT measurements similar to 45-year-old adults. These findings show a cause for concern. Obese children have been found to have stiff aortas. The aorta is the largest artery in the body which delivers blood from the heart to the network of arteries in the body. Proper blood flow through this vessel is very critical. A stiff aorta usually results in increased blood pressure and increased risk of cardiac and vascular diseases. Stiff blood vessels are caused by inflammation in the blood vessels; as the body tries to heal itself, it lays down calcium to heal the inflammation, thereby decreasing elasticity.

The elasticity of blood vessels is very important to blood pressure. Blood pressure is the amount of force that blood exerts on the walls of blood vessels as it passes through them. There are two pressures measured with blood pressure. **Systolic** is a measure of the pressure that occurs while the heart is beating (the top number) and **diastolic** is the pressure while the heart is relaxed (the bottom number). The heart is a pump forcing blood throughout the body. Pulse is used to measure the speed the heart is pumping. When the heart contracts an increased amount of pressure is needed to move the blood (systolic). Between heart beats, it is relaxed and filling with blood (diastolic). Tight constricted blood vessels require the heart to work harder, thus increasing blood pressure and pulse. On the other hand, dilated blood vessels allow the blood to flow easier through the vascular system, decreasing how hard the heart has to work and therefore lowering blood pressure and pulse. Increasing the diameter of a blood vessel by 15% doubles the blood flow, allowing more oxygen to reach the body. High blood pressure is known as hypertension. Normal blood pressure is 120/80 mmHg. Stage 1 Hypertension gives a diastolic reading of 90 – 99 mmHg and systolic reading of 140 – 159 mmHg. Stage 2 Hypertension gives a diastolic reading of ≥ 100 mmHg and a systolic reading of ≥ 160 mmHg. Elevated blood pressure increases the risk of heart attack and stroke. As blood vessels become scarred, hardened and less elastic, they are more likely to become blocked or rupture. It is important to maintain a balanced blood pressure. Having a systolic blood pressure below 90 mmHg is considered hypotension and can be life-threatening in severe cases.

The importance of circulation to health is not something that should be overlooked. Maintaining proper blood flow to the body is essential to preventing diseases in the peripheral, cerebral and cardiovascular systems. Reducing risk factors that can inhibit blood movement should be considered as early as childhood.

References:
1. http://www.nlm.nih.gov/medlineplus/peripheralarterialdisease.html
2. http://www.epodiatry.com/poor-circulation.htm
3. http://www.godswaynutrition.com/disorders/poorcirculation.html
4. http://www.medindia.net/news/view_news_main.asp?x=15885#ixzz1VOq SFKYw
5. http://www.cardiachealth.ca/templates/content/pages/didyouknow5.html
6. Le, J., Zhang, D., Menees, S., Chen, J., Raghuveer, G. (2010). "Vascular age" is advanced in children with atherosclerosis-promoting risk factors. Circ Cardiovasc Imaging, (3)8-14.
7. Raghuveer, G. (2010). Lifetime cardiovascular risk of childhood obesity. Am J Clin Nutr, 91(suppl):1514S-9S.

Genetics

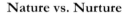

Nature vs. Nurture

The influential role of genetics on disease has often been a controversial topic. The human genome project which began in 1990 attempted to sequence all the genes in the human body. A common goal of the project included identifying genetic variants that could potentially increase the likelihood of developing disease. The many ethical issues and potential outcomes surrounding this topic stirred much debate in the media and even contributed to the making of the Hollywood movie Gattaca. The field of genetics and the many directions it can take has also played a role in agriculture. The first genetically modified food was introduced on the market in 1996. The long-term consequences of genetically modified foods are a growing concern. The introduction of foreign genes into food plants may have unexpected and negative impacts on human health. Today many products used daily are genetically modified, in particular soybean, corn, canola, rice and cotton seed oil.

Genetics can definitely play a role in health however, it is important to note the difference between genetic disorders and genetic tendencies. Genetic disorders are the result of abnormal genes, chromosomes or DNA mutations. These alterations can be present before birth, can be inherited from parents and can occur later in life. Cystic fibrosis, Tay Sach's disease, Down's Syndrome, Klinefelter syndrome and Turner syndrome are all examples of disorders that are present from birth. These DNA modifications inevitably have an effect on growth and development.

Certain human viruses and bacteria have the ability to alter human DNA. In order to replicate, these particular microorganisms are absorbed and reproduced inside human cells. In some cases, these foreign invaders can insert their DNA into ours. For example, the *herpes* virus can remain inside the cell and interfere with the cell's normal processes long after the initial infection. The portion of the *herpes* viral genome that is left over can reactivate the virus later in life causing painful Shingles. In cases like these, genes have a direct impact on the presence of a disease.

Genetic tendencies, on the other hand, do not guarantee that you will acquire the disease. Many people have a family health history with a chronic disease or health condition, such as heart disease, diabetes, high blood pressure or high cholesterol. Having a family member with this condition suggests a higher risk for developing that disease, although genetics is not the only factor that needs to be considered. Lifestyle, environment, behaviour and diet all play a key role in health and disease. Genes are very susceptible to the environment. Ultraviolet light, nuclear radiation, heavy metals and certain chemicals can damage DNA. There have also been correlations made between microwaves and mobile phone use with genetic damage.

Genetic disorders are often confused with genetic tendencies. While it is true that inheritance can play a role in the risk of developing a disease, the presence of environmental and lifestyle factors contribute significantly to determining whether you will actually develop the disease in the future.

References:
1. http://www.cdc.gov/genomics/public/index.htm
2. http://www.geneticsofpregnancy.com/Encyclopedia/The_risk_of_transmitt ing_common_diseases.aspx?pid=28&cid=49
3. http://www.csa.com/discoveryguides/gmfood/overview.php
4. Virella, G. Microbiology and Infectious Disease. 3rd edit. Williams & Wilkins. Baltimore, Maryland, 1997.

Hormones

It's a tight rope

The endocrine system is the complex glandular system in your body comprised of: the pituitary, pineal, thyroid, thymus, adrenal, pancreas, ovary and testes. These glands produce chemical messengers, known as hormones that travel through the bloodstream to tissues and organs. Hormones are essential to regulating body processes including growth and development, metabolism, digestion, breathing, blood circulation, body temperature, reproduction, sexual function and mood. Hormones control the way you respond to your environment and provide the proper amount of energy necessary for the body.

The endocrine system can become impaired and lead to an overall imbalance. Hormones are extremely potent and cause drastic changes in cells. A slight excess or deficiency may result in a variety of conditions including acne, migraines, depression, weight gain, diabetes, menopause, osteoporosis, polycystic ovarian syndrome, thyroid disorders, growth delays, infertility and more.

Keeping hormones in check is a delicate balancing act. Stress, infection and changes in your blood's fluid and electrolyte balance also influence hormone levels. Natural hormones are not the only factors that affect the endocrine system. Pharmaceutical hormones administered for birth control, fertility and hot flashes also cause a disruption. Synthetic hormones are not exactly the same as natural hormones; they contain an extra side chain (so they can be patented) that is not found in naturally occurring hormones. This molecular change in the pharmaceutical drug creates a stronger affinity for the receptor sites on cells. In other words, they will bind for longer than the hormones produced by our bodies, activating the tissue for an extended period of time. In addition, these synthetic hormones will not only flood receptor sites, they may affect the binding sites of many other hormones that they should not bind to. The endocrine system requires a delicate balance and therefore more potent hormones are not actually better. The over-flooded receptor sites stop responding and no longer provide essential functions to the body. This can lead to serious alterations and possibly disease. For example, synthetic hormones in the birth control pill can activate estrogen sensitive tissue. These excess estrogens stimulate cell division and growth resulting in endometrioses or even breast cancer.

Chemical compounds in the environment mimic hormones once they get inside the body. Low dosages of estrogenic chemicals can irreversibly alter programming in female reproductive cycles, playing a further role in endocrine conditions. For example, plastic products release chemicals that act like estrogen in the human body (http://www.sciencedaily.com/releases/2009/03/090326100

714.htm). Hormone disruptors, found in our food, also mimic natural hormones and create imbalances. Meat and dairy have the highest levels of persistent hormone disruptors. Estrogenic hormones are given to cattle, pigs and poultry so they grow bigger and fatter faster. One in particular, Bovine Growth Hormone (BGH) is given to cows to increase milk production and may be shown to increase the risk of breast cancer in humans.

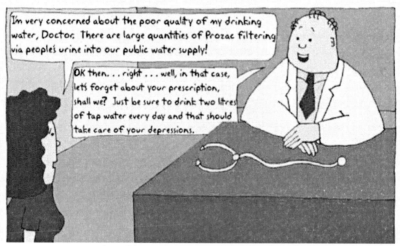

http://www.thenhf.com/article.php?id=99

An interesting report from the U.S. Geological Survey and Department of Environmental Protection revealed that 42-79% of the male smallmouth bass from the Potomac River in Washington DC, have started producing eggs. Similar results have been found throughout Europe. In Colorado, female fish have been having trouble reproducing. Left over estrogen from humans, cattle, pigs and poultry is disrupting the fish's reproduction and feminizing males.

Our water system is contaminated with pharmaceutical drugs. The Canadian federal government's first study of drinking water found traces of common painkillers, anti-cholesterol drugs and the antidepressant Prozac. After a person has taken drugs, active byproducts of these substances are released into sewage through urine or feces. These metabolites are not completely removed during the sewage-treatment process. Drug contaminated wastewater can enter groundwater or surface water and eventually be consumed by people. The National Water Research Institute for Health and Environment Canada found 9 different drugs in water samples taken near 20 drinking water treatment plants across southern Ontario. Accumulation of these metabolites disrupts hormones and affects the endocrine system.

Bioidentical hormones are used in attempts to correct an imbalance. These are made from botanical plants such as soy. These products are identified by the human body as being chemically identical to their natural hormones. In other words, the body responds to the hormones as if it were produced from the body rather than as a foreign substance.

We are continuously exposed to chemicals and hormones in our environment and even in our diet. Accumulation of these products in the body can easily alter the function of the endocrine system. It is important to be aware of how hormones, both natural and synthetic, can influence future health problems.

References:
1. http://www.nlm.nih.gov/medlineplus/endocrinediseases.html
2. http://hormonesbalancing.com/
3. http://www.hormone.org/Public/conditions.cfm
4. Berkson, D.L. Hormone Deception: How Everyday Food and Products are Disrupting Your Hormones and How to Protect Yourself and Your Family. Contemporary Books, Chicago, Illinois. 2000.
5. http://www.npr.org/2011/03/02/134196209/study-most-plastics-leach-hormone-like-chemicals
6. http://www.thenhf.com/article.php?id=99
7. http://news.nationalgeographic.com/news/2009/11/091112-drinking-water-cocaine/

Structural Damage

Not working the way it used to

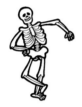

Damage to the body can occur in a variety of ways: accidental injuries, falls, sport injuries, repetitive strain or overuse. Other forms of trauma can all lead to misalignment of the joints, muscles, nerves, organs and the spine. This form of stress on the body often requires immediate attention especially because of the associated pain and immobility from the injury. Causes of an injury may often be obvious, although there are cases where the source of the structural damage is less visible.

Repetitive movements can gradually wear down your body and cause micro-trauma. This form of injury tends to occur slowly. Usually the individual becomes accustomed to the discomfort or has learned to ignore the changes until the effects are finally painful enough to seek out treatment. Continuous wear and tear to muscles, tendons and ligaments over time can lead to compensation from the surrounding structures. Poor posture, bad sleeping habits, improper lifting or carrying of heavy loads, inferior workstation habits or design and exercise are only a few of the many causes of chronic tension and structural damage.

Chemical and emotional causes can also affect the body. Poor diet, drugs, alcohol and chemical toxins in the food, air or water can decrease the body's ability to function and adapt to stressors. Inadequate stress management affects physical health and decreases immune function. The combination of these factors makes the body more susceptible to injury and disease.

Poor sleeping habits are one of the most common causes of misalignment, especially to the spine. Sleeping on your stomach or with too many pillows, places continual stress on the cervical spine and causes a shift of the vertebrae. Serious illness and disability may result as many important nerves that supply the entire body travel through the cervical spine.

The causes of stress to the body may vary but the results are largely the same: gradual displacement of the joint or vertebrae resulting in dysfunction to the body. Pain, tenderness, stiffness, decreased mobility, numbness or tingling are merely a few symptoms of structural damage to the body. Massage therapy can help relieve muscle spasms and tight muscles that cause pain and pull joints or vertebrae out of place. Chiropractors and Naturopathic Doctors can remove subluxations and misalignments of the spine, however if the pain persists and you need ongoing treatment then the problem may be from nerves, muscles, tendons or ligament damage. Alternative therapies such as prolotherapy (for tendons and

131

ligaments), Neural treatment (for nerves), Trigger Point Injection (for muscles) and Platelet Rich Plasma (tendons, ligaments and joints) may need to be considered in order to repair the damage.

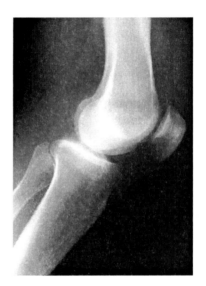

References:

1. http://www.demosschiropractic.com/vertebral-subluxation.cfm
2. http://www.desitwist.com/general-knowledge/poor-sleeping-posture-may-cause-spinal-misalignment-18496.html
3. http://www.dcdoctor.com/pages/rightpages_allaboutchiro/subluxations.html

Weak and Diseased Organs

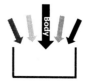

When an organ plays out of tune

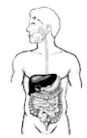

The human body is composed of several vital organ systems that work together in unison for our daily function. Numerous lifestyle factors and environmental exposures contribute to increased burden on individual or multiple organs in the body. The excess demands placed on our organs can weaken the body, exacerbate a current condition, present as new symptoms and eventually lead to a disharmony in overall health.

Traditionally there are two schools of thought around disease and the development of symptoms. From a Western science perspective, there are 10 major organ systems found in the human body. When an organ is damaged, there should be clear symptoms and changes found in lab values or observed with diagnostic imaging. This approach is very linear; A and B causes C and D. Individual symptoms are analyzed and dissected until causal links are found to be able to make a diagnosis. Blood work should show tissue damage to the specific organ. While this approach can be effective, it may not always work in explaining your symptoms. A 1989 study revealed the inadequacies of diagnostic testing for many common complaints including fatigue, dizziness, headache, edema, back pain, insomnia, abdominal pain, etc. From the 567 complaints examined, an actual cause determined by lab testing was found in only 16 percent. Treatment was provided for 55 percent of symptoms and the outcomes were often ineffective; merely 164 of the 307 symptoms improved. The study suggests that evaluation and management of individual symptoms are not universal for each person and should be refined. Have there been occasions where you have noticed changes in your body, mood or energy yet medical doctors were not able to find a problem (all your lab values appear normal)? From a Traditional Chinese Medicine (TCM) perspective, a weakened organ displaying symptoms will often not show any changes to labs or blood work. TCM organs hold a different meaning than the mainstream medical approach.

The two schools of thought have different approaches to understanding symptoms, disease and health. The modern medical belief of health is often considered to be the absence of disease; blood work is normal therefore you are healthy. The true definition of health encompasses the body as a whole: "a state of complete physical, mental and social well-being". This definition of health was actually drafted by the World Health Organization in 1946 and still remains a subject of controversy. This view does correlate with the TCM measure of health that evolved over 5000 years. Parallels can be drawn between each view of health and their motivations for treatment. Throughout history, payment for each visit to a medical doctor was expected for eliminating the disease. In ancient times Chinese doctors were paid to keep their patients healthy and were not given payment if their patient became ill. During the Zhou Dynasty 3000 years ago, doctors wore divided into different groups according to their responsibility, *ji yi* (doctors for curing internal disease) *yan yi* (doctors for external disorders), *shou yi* (veterinary doctors) and *shi yi* (dietetic doctors). Various doctors had to undergo examinations at the end of each year, judged in terms of the effectiveness of their treatments, to determine their salary. The reward system for these examinations was: full salary for a 100% cure rate, and decreased salary based on the percentage of treatment failure. Therefore doctors were urged to improve their medical skill in order to achieve better compensation for their profession. One approach again looks at the presence of disease while the other looks at total health and the goal of attaining optimal health.

In TCM there are 5 major organ systems and 6 minor systems. Each organ system has an effect on another organ system when it becomes imbalanced. These organs do not actually refer to the specific tissue as an individual physical unit, but rather the interrelated functions associated with it. For example, damage to the Western (science) liver will show increased liver enzymes and serious changes to its structure. A weakened TCM liver may appear as changes to the eyes and vision, anger and emotional frustration, menstrual difficulties or digestive difficulties. In TCM, the organ systems are all connected and more than one organ can be used in treatment. In addition, the weak and diseased organs also hold different meanings. In Western medicine, these terms are often used interchangeably; diseased organs are weak and understood to lead to illness. In TCM, weakened organs can lead to a disharmony in health although these organs may or may not be diseased. A diseased organ alternatively may not appear weak. For example, a cancerous lesion found in the liver may not display decreased function as the organ system may have compensated. Recognizing these relationships in organ function is important in understanding organ pathology. Chinese methodology was developed over many thousands of years by considering the person as a whole. Therefore each sign and symptom is used to establish a complete picture before a diagnosis and treatment plan is made. The root cause of all the symptoms is treated in TCM instead of chasing individual symptoms.

Our daily lifestyle and environment can place a great deal of physical, mental and emotional strain on the body. While there are two approaches to understanding organ systems and their relationships to symptoms, multiple diseases can result when organ function begins to weaken or is damaged from increased demand. It is important to maintain optimal health to strengthen the immune system and protect the body from developing pathology.

References:

1. Kaptchuk, T. The Web that has no Weaver. Congdon & Weed, Inc. New York, New York. 1983.
2. Kroenke, K. & Mangelsdorff, AD. Common symptoms in ambulatory care: incidence, evaluation, therapy and outcome. American Journal of Medicine. 1989; 86(3):262-6.
3. http://www.medizin-ethik.ch/publik/historical_overview.htm

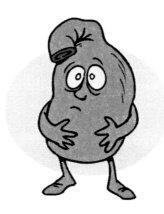

What do Labs Mean?

Labs

Laboratory tests often require a sample of your blood, urine or body tissue, to help determine what you may be at risk for, diagnose or rule out a disease, monitor particular chemistries in your body and track progress of treatments. Below is a list of some standard and some additional comprehensive tests to help explain what these tests are and what they could indicate.

At NaturoMedic.com we can provide requisitions for the following labs in Ontario, however, please note that they are not covered by OHIP or private health insurance providers.

Standard Lab Work

Lab	Description
Complete Blood Count (CBC)	There are many components tested on a routine CBC, some of the main areas are: WBC: White blood cell count measures the amount of leukocytes in the blood. There are different types of white blood cells, including T-cells and B-cells. Increased amounts usually indicate infection. RBC: Red blood cell count measures the amount of erythrocytes in the blood. RBC contains hemoglobin, responsible for carrying and transporting oxygen. Low levels usually suggest hemorrhage, anemia, and chronic illness. Hemoglobin: the molecule in the RBC that carries oxygen from the lungs to the body and returns carbon dioxide. Low levels found in anemia, severe hemorrhage, nutritional deficiency etc... Platelet count: Platelets, also known as thrombocytes, are the smallest cell-like structures in the blood that are important for blood clotting, plugging damaged blood vessels and wounds. Increased amounts can occur with trauma, rheumatoid arthritis and malignancies. Low levels can suggest hemorrhage, anemia or result from cancer chemotherapy.
Cholesterol and Lipid Panel	Total cholesterol: Cholesterol is an important fat required for hormone production and healthy cells. Cholesterol testing is used to identify patients at risk for heart disease. Elevated cholesterol is usually the result of high amount of LDL cholesterol. LDL cholesterol: often referred to as "bad cholesterol" can deposit in blood vessels, clogging arteries and leading to atherosclerosis. An elevated value can suggest poor blood sugar regulation, eating food high in fat and increased risk for heart disease. HDL cholesterol: known as the "good cholesterol" protects arteries by removing cholesterol from the tissues and transporting it back to the liver for excretion. High values reduce your risk of heart disease however abnormally elevated levels can indicate liver disease. Triglycerides: free fats in the body produced by the liver and used as a storage source of energy. Excess amounts are deposited into fatty tissues, increasing the risk for heart disease.

Ferritin	Measure of available **iron stores**. Elevated levels indicate inflammation linked to heart disease, high blood pressure, diabetes and cancer or can occur with hemachromatosis. Low levels in anemia.
Glucose	Measures the level of your blood sugar. Fasting high levels suggest diabetes and low levels can indicate hypoglycemia. May also be used to monitor diabetes.
Hemoglobin A1C	Measures **blood sugar control** over the past three months. A high value can indicate pre-diabetic or diabetes.
Insulin	Hormone released by the pancreas to assist transportation of sugar into cells. Elevated levels suggest not balancing sugar, prediabetic condition or diabetes. Low amounts have been found with hypoglycemia.
C-reactive Protein (CRP)	A non-specific marker to diagnose **inflammation or acute infection**. Very elevated levels may suggest recent injury or tissue damage. Slightly elevated can suggest low-grade inflammation that can lead to chronic degenerative conditions (arthritis, heart disease, cancer).
Kidney Function Tests	Creatinine-blood: Breakdown product of muscle that is excreted entirely by the kidneys. High values indicate poor kidney function and low values may result from decreased muscle mass or debilitation. Blood Urea Nitrogen (BUN): Urea is the end product of protein metabolism formed in the liver and excreted by the kidneys. BUN measures function of both the kidney and the liver. Elevated levels may suggest kidney disease, urinary obstruction etc... although decreased amounts have been found in liver failure, malnutrition and pregnancy. Glomerular Filtration Rate (GFR): measures how well the kidneys are filtering creatinine. Urine levels of creatinine are used to calculate GFR. Elevated levels may occur with exercise and pregnancy. Decreased values suggest impaired kidney function.
Electrolytes	Provide information on acid-base balance and hydration status.
Protein	Uric Acid: Breakdown product of purines found in food and is excreted by the kidneys. Elevated levels in gout. Albumin: Main protein in the blood (60%) formed by the liver. Important to maintain water flow in and out of the blood (osmotic pressure). Low levels can suggest malnourishment Globulin: Proteins found in the blood, produced by the liver
Liver Function Tests	ALT (Alanine aminotransferase): Liver enzyme released into the blood with injury or disease to the liver. Elevated amounts with liver damage, liver disease, hepatitis, cirrhosis or exposure to toxic substances. AST (Aspartate aminotrasferase): An enzyme produced in the liver and heart. Usually measured with ALT and bilirubin to diagnose and monitor liver disease. Elevated AST/ALT ratio is found with alcoholic cirrhosis, liver congestion and metastatic live tumour. GGT (Gamma-glutamyl transferase): Liver enzyme that measures irritation and inflammation of the liver from drugs, alcohol, gallstones and gallbladder disease, and pesticide exposure. Bilirubin: A yellowish pigment produced in the metabolism of RBCs. Used to determine whether a liver or gallbladder problem exists.
Thyroid Panel	TSH (Thyroid-stimulating hormone): hormone released by the brain and tells the thyroid how hard to work. When levels are elevated, the

	thyroid is not working hard enough suggesting hypothyroidism. A low reading indicates that the thyroid is working normally or too hard as in hyperthyroidism.
	T4 (Thyroxine): hormone secreted by the thyroid in reaction to TSH. In some cases both total T4 and free T4 (the amount available for tissues) are measured. Elevated amounts are found in hyperthyroid states and low amounts in hypothyroid states.
	T3 (Triiodothryonine): the active form of the thyroid hormone produced with T4 once the thyroid is stimulated by TSH. Generally below normal amounts are found in hypothyroid states and elevated in hyperthyroid conditions.

Comprehensive Lab Work

Lab	Description
Glutathione	Major detoxifying protein and antioxidant. Low levels in chronic disease and toxin exposure. Elevated amounts with alcohol, smoking, recent toxic exposure substance.
Omega 6/3 ratio	Measure the ratio inflammatory fat (omega 6) versus healthy anti-inflammatory fats (omega-3)
Vitamin D	Hormone found to be dangerously low in majority of Canadians as it can be synthesized in the body from sun exposure. Vitamin D has been shown to increase energy, prevent colds and flu, reduce the risk of heart disease, cancer and lower blood pressure.
Vitamin B12	Important in cell reproduction, energy and conversion of homocysteine. Low levels of B12 can result in higher amounts of homocysteine which increases the risk of atherosclerosis and heart disease.

Chapter 6

Disease Causing Factors: Mind

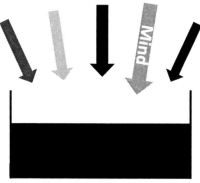

139

Sleep

Not a waste of time

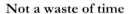

Adequate sleep is necessary not only for daily function but for optimal health and wellness. Sleep disturbances can include: difficulties falling asleep, awakening throughout the night, sleep deprivation and sleep apnea (a sleep disorder characterized by pauses in breathing during sleep). We have all experienced the bad mood, fatigue or lack of focus following a poor night's sleep. Insufficient sleep on a regular basis is associated with long-term health consequences.

Chronic sleep deprivation may affect metabolism and lead to weight gain. People who habitually sleep less than six hours per night are more likely to have a higher body mass index (BMI) than people who sleep eight hours a night. During sleep, our body secrets hormones that control energy, metabolism, appetite and glucose processing. For example, cortisol levels rise with poor sleep leading to increased appetite and deposition of fat around the abdominal area. The gain in weight ultimately results in elevated insulin levels, a hormone that regulates glucose and promotes fat storage, which can increase the risk of developing diabetes.

Alterations in one's sleep pattern causes an imbalance of hormone levels including leptin and ghrelin. Leptin is responsible for alerting the brain when the stomach is full while ghrelin stimulates appetite. An inadequate amount of sleep lowers leptin and increases ghrelin causing food cravings to occur shortly after a meal and adding to excess consumption of calories. The combined effect on the metabolism from these two important hormones lead to further complications including obesity, type II diabetes, high blood pressure, heart disease and a shortened life expectancy.

Chronic sleep issues have been correlated with depression, anxiety and decreased memory function. Memory consolidation is a process that occurs during sleep and ensures that new memories are stored. Impatience, irritability, decreased concentration and lowered immune function typically occur following lack of sleep. It is important to maintain a proper balance of sleep per night as too much sleep can also lead to poor health.

Diet and certain lifestyle factors can affect sleep. For example, caffeine in coffee, tea and soft drinks can block receptors that trigger sleep for up to 6-8 hours. Other stimulants can keep you awake. Nicotine can cause lighter sleep. Alcohol is a sedative that can prevent deep sleep or reaching rapid eye movement (REM) sleep (the dream stage of sleep). Large meals or exercise prior to bedtime can create difficulties in falling asleep. Conversely, exercise at night delays the release of melatonin which helps the body to fall asleep, while exercise during the day can actually improve the quality of sleep. Bright lights, television, computer and other noise distractions affect a good night's sleep. An uncomfortable mattress and pillow decreases your ability to fall and stay asleep.

There is a clear relationship between sleep and our ability to function during the day. The implications of getting sufficient sleep on a regular basis are essential to health and healing. Research suggests that 8 hours of sleep is optimal.

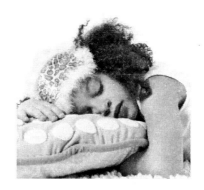

References:
1. Harvard Medical School Health Publications:
    http://www.health.harvard.edu/press_releases/importance_of_sleep_and_h
    ealth
2. US Department of Health and Human Services:
    http://www.nhlbi.nih.gov/health/public/sleep/healthy_sleep.pdf

Social Network

More than just logged on

In the past few years, the media has placed more attention on the mind, body and spirit connection with your health. Your health is affected by more than just physical aspects; your social life in fact can have a large impact on mortality and longevity. Many do not realize how important relationships are to the quality of their lives.

Your daily interactions with others provide a way to release stress, contributing to a healthier immune system and overall better health. When you have someone to talk to about your terrible boss or your financial concerns, they can sympathize, provide solutions or offer advice. What you may not realize is that all these factors can lead to improved health and a longer life expectancy. Genetically, there are 209 socially regulated genes identified in the human body, including those involved in the immune system, cell proliferation and responses to stress. You will discover as you read the following insights how important social interactions are to our body.

Numerous studies have shown that having few relationships or weak social ties can be dangerous to your health. A recent article from Brigham Young University reported that social connections improve the odds of survival by 50 percent. A poor social life was equivalent to: smoking 15 cigarettes a day, being an alcoholic, being twice as harmful as obesity and more harmful than not exercising. The health impact of social networks on mortality has actually been studied since the 70s. A nine-year follow-up study of 6,928 adults in California showed that people who lacked social and community ties had increased mortality compared to those with more extensive contacts. A similar fourteen-year follow-up study of 1,752 adults found that having more social contacts meant delayed mortality, particularly with cardiovascular risk. The feeling of loneliness was associated with increased cardiovascular death, especially in males.

Loneliness and isolation have been cited as causing many adverse health outcomes including increased risk of developing inflammatory disease (autoimmune disorders, rheumatoid arthritis, etc.), low-grade peripheral inflammation, cardiovascular disease, systolic blood pressure changes and more susceptibility to developing colds. There is clear evidence of the importance of social connections with family, friends, neighbours and colleagues to our health. Nevertheless, these interactions are changing with the major influence of online social networks.

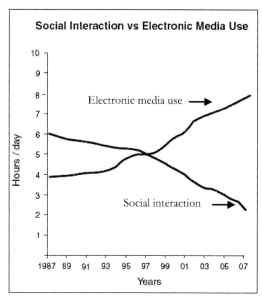

Figure 1. Hours per day of face-to-face social interaction declines as use of electronic media increases. These trends are predicted to increase (data abstracted from a series of time-use and demographic studies).

http://azureim.files.wordpress.com/2009/02/sigmanbiologist2009.pdf

There has been a steady decline in the amount of face to face social interactions with the rise of electronic media use. Internet, email and text messaging do ultimately create many advantages and conveniences for communication. At the same time they are also changing the way we interact with each other. The Internet Paradox was a study completed over a decade ago with 73 families. The researchers concluded that increased use of the internet was associated with a decline in communication between family members in the house, a decline in the size of their social circle and increases in their levels of depression and loneliness. This study was published in 1998 and predated the development of Facebook, Twitter, MySpace, instant messaging, etc. The authors did in fact complete a follow-up report in 2001. The Internet Paradox Revisited was more optimistic about the internet actually increasing social interactions. While it is true that you may have more connections the more friends you have on Facebook or the more followers you have on twitter, but the face-to-face contact is what appears to be the health determining factor. Dr. Aric Sigman suggests that the lack of real social networking involving personal interaction may have biological effects. He proposes that this could alter the way genes work, decrease immune response, lower hormone levels, diminish arterial function and influence mental performance. These changes can lead to increased risk of cancer, stroke, heart disease and dementia. The face-to–face interaction is the critical factor to your health.

At NaturoMedic.com we are not opposed to social networking technology. On the contrary, we believe the collaborative opportunities and the ability to stay in touch with distant friends and relatives is quite valuable. We would however seek to make you aware of the implications to your health. Social media have actually been the subject of extensive research over the past couple of years; both positive and negative results have been determined. Improvements in self-esteem, strengthening of relationship ties and creating opportunities of conversation for those with low social skills have been found as a benefit. Alternatively, it may also cause depression, trigger eating disorders and split up marriages. According to a new study in 2009 from Loyola University, Facebook is cited in 1 out of 5 divorces and is the number one source for online evidence in over half of divorce cases. We doubt this was Mark Zuckerberg's, Facebook's developer, intention.

So the next time you are debating whether to go for a run, call a friend, visit a neighbour or keep a dinner date with your spouse, consider all the health benefits you may receive.

References:
1. http://www.plosmedicine.org/article/info:doi/10.1371/journal.pmed.100003 16
2. http://www.dailymail.co.uk/health/article-1149207/How-using-Facebook-raise-risk-cancer.html#ixzz1eYBlELnV
3. BerkMan L & Syme L. Social Networks, host resistance and mortality: a nine-year follow-up study of Alameda county residents. Oxford Journals, 1979. http://aje.oxfordjournals.org/content/109/2/186.short
4. Olsen R., Olsen J. Gunner-Svensson F. & Waldstom B. Social networks and longevity. A 14 year follow-up study among elderly in Denmark. Elsevier 2002.
5. http://www.sciencedirect.com/science/article/pii/0277953691902355
6. http://www.theappgap.com/how-does-social-networking-affect-your-health-and-well-being.html
7. Sigman A. Well Connected?:The Biological Implications of 'Social Networking. Biologist. Volume 56 Number 1, pages 14-20. 19th February 2009. http://azureim.files.wordpress.com/2009/02/sigmanbiologist2009.pdf
8. http://www.everydayhealth.com/healthy-living/0406/the-facebook-effect-good-or-bad-for-your-health.aspx

Stress Management

Fight, Flight or Freeze

What is stress exactly?

Stress comes in many forms. It can be defined as anything real or perceived that causes your body to react. This reaction is your body's attempt to cope with a challenge, frustration or threat. It begins in the nervous system and then cascades to every facet of the body. Stress affects your thoughts, your digestion, your hormones, your blood pressure and your sleep…essentially everything in your body.

These real or perceived forms of stress can be major or minor. Major stresses could include a death in the family, coping with a chronic illness, moving, a wedding, loss of a job or starting a new job, etc. Both positive and negative events can cause a great deal of stress. For some even minor occurrences like a misunderstanding with a co-worker or being late for an appointment can cause major stress. How your body deals with these events depends on what sort of coping mechanisms you are using and how resilient your body is at that time.

The body's natural response to stress is to activate the sympathetic nervous system, which triggers the "fight, flight or freeze response" as if you were being stalked or attacked by a predator. You breathe faster, your heart beats stronger, blood moves away from your organs and into your skeletal muscles to increase strength and speed. All this is meant to give you a better chance to survive a predator attack. Most of us are not in a life or death situation on a daily basis when stress occurs. All of the these physiological responses still occur, making us feel anxious, irritated, jittery, sweaty and as if our hearts are going to beat out of our chests. If your body is reacting to things continuously, it will eventually have a negative impact. In the stress response, your body produces hormones like adrenaline and cortisol while simultaneously decreasing the production of beneficial hormones like DHEA (anti-stress and anti-aging hormone).

The implications of a long-term, highly stressed state are vast. The heart, digestion and immune system are commonly affected. Do you have high blood pressure, heart palpitations, irritable bowel or heartburn? Do you have headaches, low energy or difficulty sleeping? Are you prone to getting sick? In any of these situations stress can be the root cause.

What can you do to increase your resiliency to stress?

Improve your sleep habits

Regular aerobic exercise

A balanced diet of non-processed foods

Diaphragmatic breathing (Inhale-abdomen expands, Exhale-abdomen contracts. Breathing only through the nose)

NaturoMedic.com also offers several services to improve your ability to handle stress including:
HeartMath
Mental Reprogramming Technique
Botanical Medicines and Chinese Herbal Patents
Diet and Lifestyle Counseling
Nutritional Supplements
Homeopathic Medicine

Some of the ways Chronic Stress Affects Your Health

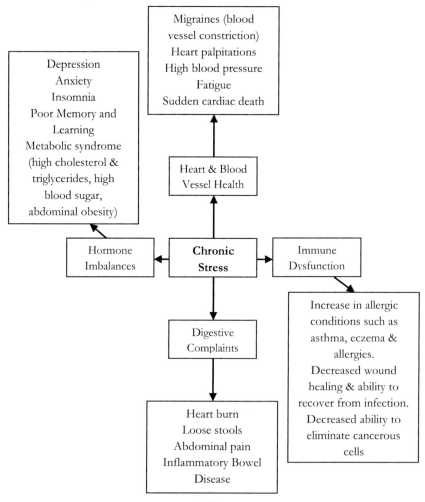

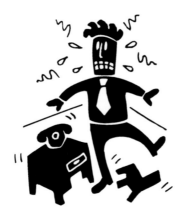

References:

1. R A, N P, DA P, JF S. Social interactions, stress, and immunity. Immunol Allergy Clin North Am. 2009;29:285-293.

2. ND D, L X, KE R, Jr MGD. Stress and allergic diseases. Immunol Allergy Clin North Am. 2011;31:55-68.

3. Godbout JP R G. Stress-induced immune dysregulation: implications for wound healing, infectious disease and cancer. Journal Of Neuroimmune Pharmacology: The Official Journal Of The Society On Neuroimmune Pharmacology. 2006;1

4. JE G, LM C, JK K-G. Stress, age, and immune function: toward a lifespan approach. J Behav Med. 2006;29:389-400.

5. SA R. Hypercortisolism as a potential concern for submariners. Aviation, Space, and Environmental Medicine. 2010;81:1114-1122.

6. PJ R. Perplexing Immune Responses To Stress. Health And Stress. The Newsletter of The American Institute of Stress. 2008;9:1-12.

7. FT, JM, IE. Psychoneuroimmunology. Dermatologic Therapy. 2008; 21:22–31.

Finances

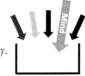

No complaint is more common than that of a scarcity of money.
— Adam Smith

We have all heard the lyrics from that popular song "money makes the world go round." We may not like it, but money and finances are a necessary part of life.

Since the recent recession experienced by Canada and the USA, a number of surveys and studies have been conducted around the topic of finances. A 2012 Canadian Payroll Association survey discovered that 47% of Canadians live from pay cheque to pay cheque. A health-related survey by Sun Life Financial showed that 72% of those asked said they were experiencing "excessive" levels of anxiety over financial concerns. An article published in the Globe and Mail in November 2012 had this to say about Canadians and our finances: "so much of money stress is caused by overspending, which is the toughest financial challenge in Canadian society today". There is no doubt that money is on people's minds.

We all know that one's financial situation can be a stressor, but can it actually make us sick? Several studies have now shown the negative effects worrying about money (or lack thereof) can have on a person's health. Research has implicated that high levels of stress about debt is twice as likely to cause a heart attack. A US poll carried out by the Associated Press indicated an increased percentage of digestive tract problems, headaches or migraines and depression in those with high stress levels over finances. Reportedly, highly stressed individuals were 65% more likely to suffer from back pain and muscle tension than those with low stress. Financial worries have also been linked to other stress-related illnesses such as ulcers and anxiety.

Another interesting survey discovered that a majority of Americans would rather gain weight than take on more debt. Apparently 78% of those asked would rather gain ten pounds than accept $10,000 in more debt. Thankfully, we at NaturoMedic.com do not see the situation as an either/or choice. It is no wonder that the Bible had so much to say on the topic of money. According to histories oldest book, "the love of money is the root of all kinds of evils."

Everyone has heard stories about the spinster who squirreled away so much wealth that the family was shocked at the reading of her extensive will. And it is not uncommon today to read in the paper about a bankrupt millionaire with a huge mansion. The team at NaturoMedic.com recommends neither of these approaches, but a balance in the middle.

One successful debt management strategy was created by Dave Ramsey, a US radio show host and author. Ramsey travels widely in North America teaching a variety of financial skills to all ages. His radio show often features amazing testimonies of people who developed a strategy and budget for their money and are now reaping the benefits of working toward a goal. Ramsey has helped thousands of people dig their way out of debt and build solid financial foundations for themselves and their families over the years. Suze Orman's (as seen on Oprah) is another effective strategy. Alternatively one can perform internet search for other debt management programs.

The team at NaturoMedic.com desires to see our patients wisely managing their resources and living without the strain of financial burdens. Own money; do not let it own you.

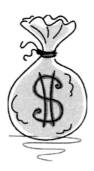

References:
1. http://www.brainyquote.com/quotes/topics/topic_money.html
2. http://www.theglobeandmail.com/globe-investor/personal-finance/household-finances/money-stress-catches-up-with-canadians/article5221810/
3. http://www.businessnewsdaily.com/2419-money-worry-health.html
4. http://www.webmd.com/balance/features/the-debt-stress-connection
5. http://www.businessnewsdaily.com/2195-weight-gain-debt.html
6. http://www.daveramsey.com/
7. 1 Timothy 6:10

Work

Find a job you like and you add five days to every week.
– H. Jackson Brown

The many hours we spend per week at a workplace, job or career can significantly contribute to our health status. One's job can be either empowering and life-giving or demoralizing and stressful. Those who regularly have to endure the latter type of environment often suffer emotional and physical harm as a result. Even relatively good working situations can cause periods of acute stress when deadlines are imminent.

Multiple studies have been conducted over the years on the relationship between jobs and stress. There is a certain amount of "good" stress that comes with every job. This type of stress is called **eu**stress (the same prefix as euphoria). Eustress is "positive" stress that motivates us and provides the incentive we often need to get things done. The excitement of riding a roller coaster or the challenge of completing a fun puzzle or competition are examples of eustress. This type of stress is healthy and is what helps us get out of the bed in the morning.

On the other hand, jobs can also cause "bad" stress, or **di**stress. This state occurs when the challenges faced from day-to-day are no longer fun; one feels buried under the weight of expectations and tension from which there seems to be no relief. This type of job stress can present itself physically in several ways. High blood pressure and rapid breathing are two common stress responses. Studies have also shown that hostile work environments and working long hours have the potential to accelerate the development of heart disease. Age can be a factor in the equation as well. A study done at the University of Utah showed that, as stressed workers aged, their blood pressure rose above average levels. Those who experience high levels of job stress succumb more often to the common cold and have to call in sick.

Job stress can also manifest in other ways. Some people find themselves constantly thinking and worrying about projects or conflicts with coworkers. Others are drained of energy and have little left over for regular exercise or healthy life habits. Often job stress leads to the development of negative coping mechanisms such as increased drinking or smoking. Overeating or a loss of appetite can also result from work-related stress. Sadly, a link has been made between high job stress and lower levels of mental health.

It seems that those in blue collar or middle-class job positions suffer from a particular type of job stress. A lack of control over one's work environment can lead to depression, anxiety and eventually emotional exhaustion (i.e. burnout). One study noted that employees with high psychological and physical job demands and little job control reported various psychosomatic and physical health complaints as well as very low job satisfaction. Prolonged or chronic stress can take its toll on the body. The development of heart disease and type II diabetes have both been linked to chronic stress.

Workplace stress can be a result of various factors. Poor management, excessively high expectations, unclear goals and guidelines, job insecurity, workplace conflict and a multitude of other things may combine to create a difficult working environment. The team at NaturoMedic.com recognizes that it may not always be possible to eliminate these stressors from one's life. "When people go to work, they should not have to leave their hearts at home". We desire to see our patients investing their time and energy in areas from which they receive satisfaction.

References:
1. http://www.quotegarden.com/jobs.html
2. http://stress.about.com/od/stressmanagementglossary/g/Eustress.htm
3. http://www.brocku.ca/health-services/health-education/stress/eustress-distress
4. http://www.apa.org/helpcenter/job-stress.aspx
5. http://stress.about.com/od/stresshealth/a/jobstress.htm
6. Betty Bender quotation

Sex

What was once a taboo subject for society in the west is no longer. Television and movies have made sex a common topic of conversation in the 21st century. Is sex a factor worth considering from a health perspective? Let us take a look.

Studies have now been conducted to evaluate the effects of sex on a person's health. According to an article published in 2009, regular sex improves health and doubles life expectancy. A survey conducted of 10,000 middle age men revealed that those who reported the highest frequency of orgasm lived twice as long as those who did not enjoy sex. Another study conducted concluded that sexual activity seems to have a protective effect on men's health.

So sex can contribute to longevity in men. Does it have specific health benefits for women too? According to recent research, it has many. One interesting finding by an MD, the founder of the PATH Medical Center in New York City, is that sex may give women healthier-looking skin. During sex, the body produces the hormone DHEA (dehydroepiandrosterone). This chemical does several good things for the body, including improving one's complexion. Another possible benefit of sex for women is increased bladder control as the muscles associated with incontinence (the pelvic floor muscles) can be exercised and strengthened during intercourse.

Sex has many other health perks across the board for both men and women. It has been proven to have a role in reducing high blood pressure and increasing circulation. Apparently those who have sex regularly are half as likely to have heart attacks and strokes as those who do not have sex at all. Sex can also be a weight loss tool because of the increased calories burned as well as the phenetylamine produced during intercourse, a hormone that regulates appetite. Having sex can even combat the common cold because the body releases an antibody during orgasm called immunoglobulin A which is known to strengthen immunity.

Sex can also be a good stress reliever. Oxytocin is a chemical that the body releases just before orgasm. This chemical aides in the secretion of endorphins which help the body relax or "chill out". Because of this, sex can be a natural remedy for insomnia. Other health benefits range from improved cognition to decreased incidences of breast cancer to increased pain tolerance.

There are also emotional health benefits to a healthy sex life. A survey of 500 Americans demonstrated that over 80% of married men and women believed a satisfying sex life was important to their individual lives and their relationship.

Almost 100% of those involved in the survey indicated that sexual enjoyment improves one's quality of life at any age. Research has also demonstrated support for the theory that regular intercourse can be linked to a decreased risk of depression. Another study concluded that consistent mutual sexual pleasure increases bonding within a relationship. It appears that sex within a healthy, stable relationship is a great tool for maintaining one's well-being.

We would be remiss not to mention the potential negative health implications of sex as well. An article published in 2011 stated that having sex during the adolescent years can have negative effects on a person's body and mood well into adulthood. Zachary Weil, from the Department of Neuroscience at Ohio State University concluded that there is a time in nervous system development when things are changing very rapidly and part of those changes are preparations for adult reproductive behaviors and physiology. There is a possibility that environmental experiences and signals could have amplified effects if they occur before the nervous system has settled down into adulthood.

Chinese medicine has stressed the importance of not having excessive sexual activity. Your essence is present at birth. It forms the material basis for the whole body and is crucial in reproduction, growth, development and maturation. Every metabolic activity consumes it; we can nourish or deplete it through our behavior and lifestyle. But once it's gone, you cannot make more. Sexual activity has been known to consume your essence, although there is a distinction between its effect on men and women. Excessive activity is less of a cause of disease in women than men. Essence plays a significant role in fertility. In men, loss of sperm implies a loss of essence and therefore excessive sexual behaviours can diminish it. On the other hand, in women, there is no corresponding loss during sexual activity as they do not lose any ova, making them less likely to develop disease.

Insufficient sexual activity also plays a role in disease according to Chinese Medicine. When sexual desire is present but does not have an outlet, pathological disease can result. *Qi* is one's life force. It can become trapped with sexual frustration and a lack of release, giving rise to various gynecological problems including dysmenorrhea. Additionally, sexual frustration will affect the emotional and mental attitude. Stagnant or blocked *Qi* can contribute to feelings of loneliness and depression. Insufficient or excessive sexual activity can therefore be a disease causing factor according to Traditional Chinese Medical views.

Of course we must point out the risks associated with having sex. Sexually transmitted diseases (STDs) are still a reality today. While there may be effective treatments for some of them, they are never welcome. The Centers for Disease Control and Prevention suggests several ways to limit the incidence of STDs. Abstinence, monogamy and proper protection (e.g. condoms) are their biggest recommendations. It is essential to know your status and your partner's with respect to STDs before engaging in sexual activity. Remember when it comes to STDs you are not just sleeping with your partner; you are possibly sleeping with what was shared between your partner and their previous relationships.

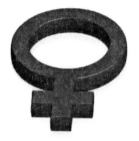 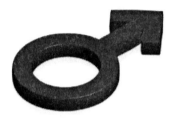

References:
1. http://www.naturalnews.com/025393_health_WHO_life.html
2. http://www.womansday.com/sex-relationships/sex-tips/8-surprising-health-benefits-of-sex-102017
3. http://www.plannedparenthood.org/files/PPFA/BenSex_07-07.pdf
4. http://www.news-medical.net/news/20111116/Sex-during-adolescence-can-have-negative-effects-on-body-and-mood-well-into-adulthood.aspx
5. http://www.cdc.gov/std/prevention/default.htm
6. http://maciociaonline.blogspot.ca/2011/07/sexual-life-in-chinese-medicine.html
7. http://www.shen-nong.com/eng/lifestyles/tcmrole_health_maintenance_habits.html

Our Subconscious

Friend or Foe?

The human brain is an elaborate and highly integrated grid consisting of billions of neurons and trillions of connections. Its capacity to acquire sensory information is exponential. The brain processes 400 billion bits of information per second, however, we are only aware of 2,000 of those. The mind takes care of all the essential items that we automatically need to respond to and yet not necessarily are conscious of. This responsibility falls mainly on the subconscious. There are a myriad of bodily functions including breathing and the pumping action of the heart that would take up all of our thinking if we were required to consciously remember to do daily. Walking, talking and driving are all programs we have deliberately created and have now become routine habits. Normal life would be impossible without the subconscious mind. Conversely, while the ability of certain stimuli to elicit physiological, behavioral and emotional responses from the subconscious can be beneficial, it also masks any negative associations we make with them.

Pavlov's dog is a popular reference often used to introduce the concept of the unconscious capabilities of the mind. The 1927 experiment was the first presentation of classical conditioning. Dogs were conditioned to respond to various stimuli such as bells, whistles and metronomes; every time the bell sounded the dog would be fed. Eventually the dog would automatically begin to salivate upon hearing the stimuli, regardless of whether food was present. Similar conditioned responses have also been demonstrated in other areas. The psychologist B.F. Skinner experimented with the idea of operant conditioning where a behavior can be modified by its consequence. Pigeons and rats made behavioral associations based on the result of their actions. Food or water was rewarded when one lever was pressed, while a shock was administered if an alternate lever was pressed. The possibility of reward may increase one's behaviour and the anticipation of punishment may decrease an undesired behavior. Negative and positive reinforcement are just a couple of examples of programs that can become ingrained in our subconscious with or without our knowledge.

The traditional view in psychology implies that emotions are a conscious action. You feel it, therefore you must be aware of it. This original belief has been challenged and it is now widely accepted that cognitive processes (emotions) can be unconscious therefore occurring without intention. In 1997, an initial attempt to demonstrate unconscious emotion was made through a series of studies by

Winkielman, Zajonc & Schwarz. Participants were asked to rate a neutral stimuli, such as inkblots, after subliminally being presented with a happy or angry face. The neutral stimuli were preferred when the participant was initially exposed to a happy face as opposed to an angry face even though both were subliminal messages. In a more recent 2008 study, scientists from the Max Planck Institute examining Human Cognitive and Brain Sciences revealed that decisions are made before we are aware of them. Researchers found micro patterns of activity in the frontopolar cortex of the brain **7 seconds** before the participant was conscious of the choice. The subconscious mind is powerful enough to alter behavior and emotion without our knowledge.

The subconscious mind is a reservoir of feelings, thoughts, urges and memories. Research shows that it takes between 90 seconds and 4 minutes to decide if you are attracted to someone. That attraction is based 7% on what is actually said, 55% on body language and 38% on the tone and speed of voice. The subconscious influences our current behavior. Furthermore, past relationship experiences may also trigger unconscious responses. A previous heated debate with a partner that provokes a strong emotional response, like anger, may become stored in the subconscious. Consequently, in a future conversation the original emotional response can immediately return. The conversation may actually have no relevance to the past debate and may simply be an innocent exchange. For instance, your partner may ask, "where are the car keys?" If the tone of voice or body language is similar to a previous argument or comes across aggressively, you may believe they are blaming you for the lost keys even though they may just be wondering if you have seen them. Regardless, the subconscious recognizes the similar tone or body language and automatically gives a similar response; defenses go up, anger rises and an argument is inevitable. The unpleasant content stored in the subconscious triggers programmed behaviors, all of which can be the source of relationship turmoil.

Difficulty sleeping may also have associations with subconscious programs. A child suddenly waking from a deep sleep in a dark room to the sound of parents fighting can be traumatic. Later in adulthood, subconscious emotions may be triggered every time they try to sleep in the dark. The slightest noise can cause them to wake. The experiences that register in the subconscious are not always a significant event, they may have occurred once or often. Potential fire or robbery are similar examples of threats to our survival that might create sleeping problems.

Physiological changes caused by unconscious programs are not only for Pavlov's dogs. They are quite applicable to humans. Infertility can be one such instance affected by the subconscious. Women sometimes spend years using numerous birth control methods to avoid conceiving a child. Unfortunately, when the time comes for wanting a child, the subconscious may still be telling the body, "nope, not going to happen". The negative experiences of other women may also have an influence on fertility; friends having difficulties getting pregnant may unconsciously inhibit their ability.

Subconscious programs can unknowingly interfere with daily life, work, relationships and health. While there is, of course, a great benefit to the power of the subconscious, the unpleasant consequences are not always desired. At NaturoMedic.com, we offer therapies to help delete these subconscious programs and correct the negative adverse reactions to previous events. These include the Mental Reprogramming Technique and BioClimate Reprogramming *(please refer to the individual sections for more information)*.

References:

1. http://www.lifecircles-inc.com/Learningtheories/behaviorism/Pavlov.html
2. http://www.simplypsychology.org/operant-conditioning.html
3. http://wiki.answers.com/Q/How much information can the brain proce ss#ixzz21drVpn7o
4. http://www.alice.id.tue.nl/references/Winkielman-Berridge-2004.pdf
5. http://exploringthemind.com/the-mind/brain-scans-can-reveal-your-decisions-7-seconds-before-you-decide
6. Chun Siong Soon, Marcel Brass, Hans-Jochen Heinze & John-Dylan Haynes. Unconscious Determinants of Free Decisions in the Human Brain. Nature Neuroscience, April 13th, 2008.
7. http://www.youramazingbrain.org/lovesex/sciencelove.htm

Chapter 7

Disease Causing Factors: Spirit

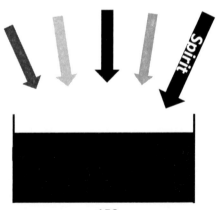

Belief: Faith and Hope

Seeing it through

As North Americans, we have become accustomed to relying on our individuality, education and internal resolve to get us through the tough times in life. If that fails, we have a number of government institutions and insurance companies to hopefully rise to the occasion in our time of need. In developing countries, individuality and education are not as preeminent as they are in North America, Europe and developed Asia. The strength of the family and the belief in a higher power take on more significant meaning. Most governments in developing countries have proven unreliable thereby reinforcing tighter family units and religious affiliations. In North America, Europe and developed Asia, we require less faith and hope, as we have a strong belief in ourselves and our ability, as shown by the general decline in religious belief and church attendance. In developing countries, the opposite is true: faith, belief and hope manifest more as conversations commonly center on the supernatural. Church attendance is much more common, as is reliance upon powers outside of oneself (e.g. the Catholic Church, Islam or spiritism). When people could not make rational (educated) sense of the events of 9/11 or more recently hurricanes Rita, Katrina and Sandy, church attendance soared. People were once again becoming dependent upon a higher power as faith in the government failed; education and individuality were not sufficient to explain these tragedies.

The power of belief, faith and hope can have on your health should not be underestimated. The connection goes beyond the institution of religion; "For as a man thinks in his heart, so is he". This of course can encompass personal spiritual views, but the capabilities of human intention have actually been studied in the area of quantum physics. There have been cases throughout the world of healers directing positive energy towards individuals suffering from disease and being able to remove the illness. Have you ever really hoped and strived for something that eventually happened? These are examples of intention. The ability of positive and negative thoughts, to affect outcomes is not something supernatural; it is a reality that has been demonstrated in science.

The quantum physicist Gary Schwartz demonstrated that direct intention can manifest as electrical and magnetic energy to produce both a visible and measureable stream of electrons. Being able to measure thought and intention has multiple applications especially when attempting to understand the strong influence it can have on actions. Early experiments connecting plants to polygraph equipment revealed that plants react when positive or negative actions towards them are intended. Cleve Backster in 1966 while working for the CIA, was the first to propose that plants are affected by human intention. His research showed plants were able to sense when a harmful thought occurred. Ongoing work on living organisms suggests that thoughts are comprised of a stream of photons and it is plausible that a plant could sense and be affected by intention signals; the plants reacted when someone just intended to do harm. Plants are not the only living organisms that can be affected by positive and negative thoughts. When you send an intention, every major physiological system in your body will be mirrored in the body of the receiver; in essence the two become one. This is evidence that our emotional responses are constantly being picked up and echoed in those close to us.

Research on the effects of thoughts has also been able to demonstrate that our bodies can anticipate and react to our future emotions before we are even consciously aware of it. In 1997, a lab at the University of Nevada monitored physiological changes in volunteers. Heart rate, blood pressure and skin conduction were measured while color photos designed to calm, arouse or upset the participant were randomly displayed. The lab discovered that physiological responses registered before the photo was shown. This was the first documented proof that our bodies unconsciously anticipate events to act out our own future emotional states. Scientists from the Max Planck Institute examining Human Cognitive and Brain Sciences revealed in 2008 that decisions are made before we are aware of them. Researchers found micro patterns of activity in the frontopolar cortex of the brain **7 seconds** before the participant was conscious of the choice. From a health perspective we know that negative thoughts or experiences can lead to physiological changes, but the idea that our body can react before we are aware that something terrible has occurred demonstrates the strong connection between the mind and body. In fact, we can further build on this to learn how to understand these reactions. Imagine the effect of avoiding harmful threats, maintaining positive thoughts and emotions and promoting optimization of health for not only ourselves but also for our family and friends. The intention that our body is sensing and that others are benefiting from is actually a form of energy that we are producing.

The ability of our thoughts to affect our bodies and those around us is quite remarkable. The power of intention can have a direct impact on your health and those close to you. A psychiatrist from California Pacific Medical Center performed a double blind experiment in 1999 with a mix of eclectic healers from America. The healers were asked to send healing thoughts to a group of HIV/AIDS patients. Each healer received a sealed packet of information about the patient and then held an intention for health for one hour a day for six days. The patient was then assigned to another healer. Eventually every patient in the treatment group was sent healing thoughts/intentions by every healer. At the end of the study each participant in the treatment group had significantly fewer HIV/AIDS defining illnesses, improved T-cell levels, fewer hospitalizations, fewer doctors' visits, fewer new illnesses, a decrease in severity of disease and a better psychological well-being than the control group. The experiment found that the intention of healing promoted the actual healing. Adversely, negative thoughts can potentially do the opposite. Studies of couples showed that the stress of reliving a previous argument delayed their healing from a wound by at least a day. Having positive intentions, beliefs and thoughts toward your health can logically contribute to improving disease symptoms.

The implications of negative thoughts can even be found in one of the world's oldest texts. In the Bible, we find multiple examples of people's disbelief impeding Jesus' ability to heal: "And because of their unbelief, he couldn't do any miracles among them except to place his hands on a few sick people and heal them". In another passage, it was not until Jesus sent everyone with negative thoughts out of the house that he was able to restore health: "When Jesus arrived at the official's home, he saw the noisy crowd and heard the funeral music. 'Get out!' he told them. 'The girl isn't dead; she's only asleep.' But the crowd laughed at him. After the crowd was put outside, however, Jesus went in and took the girl by the hand, and she stood up!" While the above examples certainly address the importance of eliminating negativity and creating a positive environment, there is an additional step that has been suggested. Positivity on its own is not enough; faith must be placed in something or someone. The 1999 experiment with eclectic healers was successful not only because of the positive intentions but also because of the healer's faith. Being positive and upbeat is merely an emotional state without any connection to a spiritual realm. The healers had a connection point to a spiritual reality. The positive atmosphere of belief must therefore be connected to that something or someone.

In the 1990s, the water experiments by Dr. Masaru Emoto, is another example of the power of thoughts. The series of trials observed the physical effect of prayer, music, words and environmental factors on the crystalline structure of frozen water. The focused intention altered the expression of the water ice crystals. Water from clear springs and water exposed to positive loving words appeared brilliant, complex and in a colorful snowflake pattern. Adversely, polluted water or water exposed to negative thoughts was asymmetrical, dull and incomplete. Dr. Emoto's work is evidence of the effect of thoughts and feelings on physical reality. It is remarkable to consider the extent intention can have on the events of our lives. The implication of the water crystal research creates awareness of how positivity can impact the earth, interpersonal and personal health.

Intention is a true energetic relationship. This is not something that only well-trained energy masters (Qigong, Tai Chi, etc.) have the power to harness; this is the same electric and magnetic energy that Gary Schwartz was able to measure from thoughts. Electric and magnetic energy are very prominent and important aspect to the planet. The Earth is one giant magnet with two poles, a North Pole and a South Pole, surrounded by a magnetic field. This geomagnetic field is affected by the solar system and geological changes on the Earth. Storms on Earth and in space can cause fluctuations to the field. Homing pigeons and dolphins are two examples of creatures that sense this energy; they use the Earth's geomagnetic field to navigate. In 1991, studies of water showed that basic signaling between molecules is not chemical but actually electromagnetic. There is evidence that natural geomagnetic fields have a pronounced effect on all cellular and chemical processes in living things. The heart is very susceptible to changes in geomagnetic fields. For example, during periods of increased activity, the viscosity of the blood increases, slowing down circulation. In fact, heart-attack rates rise and fall according to solar-cycle activity. Research has shown that a person's emotional state can also be communicated to the external environment by the electromagnetic field of the heart. On September 11th, 2001, National Oceanic and Atmospheric Administration space weather satellites that monitor the earth's geometric field (seismic activity) displayed a significant spike from a stress wave created by the global human emotion on that horrific day and for a few days after. The "global grief" of 911 caused a stress wave that was detected in space. The heart and the brain are particularly sensitive to geomagnetic fields. These fields affecting the physiology of the body are the same energy produced by thoughts.

Intention needs to be directed and is an energetic relationship involving the sun, atmosphere, earth and all living organisms. In the Old Testament God used intention to create the world: "And God said, 'Let there be light,' and there was light. Your current state of mind carries an intention that has an effect on life around you. The ability of your thoughts, beliefs, faith and hope to positively affect your health is often underestimated. This is a power that you can access daily and is something that can help revolutionize your mind, body and spirit.

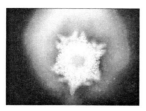

Dr. Emoto: Water crystal exposed to positive word of peace
http://www.masaru-emoto.net/english/water-crystal.html

References:
1. Backster, C. "Evidence of a Primary Perception in Plant Life." International Journal of Parapsychology.1968; 10(4): 329-48.
2. Jacques Benveniste chapter from The Field, 59
3. McTaggart, Lynn. The Intention Experiment. Free Press, New York, NY. 2007
4. Radin, D.I. "Unconscious perception of future emotions: An experiment in presentiment." Journal of Scientific Exploration, 1997; 11(2): 163-80.
5. Schwartz, G.E. and Russek, L.G. "Dynamical energy systems and modern physics". Alternative Therapies, 1997;3:46-56.
6. Sicher, F., et al. "A randomized double-blind study of the effect of distant healing in a population with advanced AIDS: Report of a small scale study." Western Journal of Medicine, 1998; 168(6): 356-63.
7. http://www.highexistence.com/water-experiment/
8. http://www.whatthebleep.com/crystals/
9. http://exploringthemind.com/the-mind/brain-scans-can-reveal-your-decisions-7-seconds-before-you-decide
10. Proverbs 23:7
11. Mark 6:5
12. Matthew 9: 23-25
13. Genesis 1:3

Forgiveness

Freedom

When you forgive, you in no way change the past –
but you sure do change the future. –Bernard Meltzer

Can unresolved relational conflicts actually affect one's health? This topic has become a hot one in recent years as research has multiplied on the emotional, mental and physical consequences of failing to forgive. Up until 1997, only 58 empirical studies had been conducted in this area. As of 2005, over 1,200 scientific papers had been published on the subject of forgiveness. "Forgiveness is being plucked out of the spiritual and theological realm and put into the psychological and physical," says psychologist and author Janis Abrahms Spring.

Research around the subject of unforgiveness has provided evidence of its negative effect on the physical body. In one study by Charlotte vanOyen Witvliet, volunteers were asked to think about a person who had mistreated or offended them. During the experiment, heart rate, blood pressure, facial tension and sweat gland activity were monitored. As people thought about the offender or the offense that had occurred, physiological responses were triggered. Heart rate and blood pressure went up and their sweat output increased. When encouraged to practice forgiveness, the physical arousal of the volunteers decreased to that of a normal resting state. In another study of unforgiveness between romantic partners with poor relationships, cortisol levels spiked when individuals were asked to think about their relationship. Cortisol is a hormone that indicates a stress response. Other studies have further shown that unforgiveness may lead to a compromised immune system.

Conversely, the practice of forgiveness has been shown to have a positive impact on physical health. In some studies, forgiveness has been correlated with a decrease in chronic back pain and depression. A study published in the Journal of Behavioural Medicine discussed the benefits of forgiveness for the heart – not surprising when we consider our own reactions to a hurt or offence. In other research, scientists have linked forgiveness to lower levels of stress hormones. One recent study led by Loren Toussaint, a psychologist from Luther College in Iowa, concluded that the physical advantages of forgiveness seem to increase with age. Their national survey showed a significant correlation between forgiving others and positive health among middle-aged and older Americans.

Psychologists have also found forgiveness to be a powerful tool in the reconciliation of marriages and families. Research seems to suggest that forgiveness lends itself to higher self-esteem, better moods and happier relationships. A study from the Personality and Social Psychology Bulletin found that forgiveness did not just affect the relationship in which the offense occurred, it also overflowed into positive behaviour toward others outside of the relationship.

We at NaturoMedic.com believe that forgiveness (or lack thereof) has spiritual ramifications, which is why we have included it in this section of the book. Everett Worthington, executive director of the Virginia foundation, A Campaign for Forgiveness Research, has discovered through various studies that people who don't have a profound faith have a more difficult time forgiving. He himself had his faith severely tested in 1995 when his mother was murdered by an intruder. Here he was – an expert in forgiveness, having authored numerous books and conducted many studies on the topic – faced with the choice to forgive a murderer or remain in bondage to the hurt and bitterness the man had caused him. Worthington's Christian faith eventually helped him to make the choice to forgive. He decided, "I knew I could be forgiven [by God]. Who am I to hold this grudge against this kid?"

The choice to forgive is really a decision to release oneself from the prison of pain and bitterness. Histories oldest book, the Bible, has a lot to say on this subject: "Then I realized that my heart was bitter, and I was all torn up inside." 'Do not seek revenge or bear a grudge." Holding a grudge and refusing to forgive those who have wronged us really hurts no one but ourselves. "If you forgive those who sin against you, your heavenly Father will forgive you."

How forgiving are you? Check out this forgiveness quiz to determine your level of forgiveness: http://www.thepowerofforgiveness.com/quiz/index.cfm.

At NaturoMedic.com, we recognize that unforgiveness can be a potential barrier to optimal health in a patient's life. We encourage our patients to practice forgiveness and also suggest methods of positive reinforcement in this process (e.g. gratitude journaling). Forgiveness is for you, not the offender. Give them a gift of forgiveness and release yourself.

"To err is human, to forgive, divine" (Alexander Pope)

References:

1. http://www.brainyquote.com/quotes/topics/topic_forgiveness.html
2. http://www.ahinternational.org/media-home/news-articles/29/204-researchers-break-down-benefits-of-forgiveness
3. http://greatergood.berkeley.edu/article/item/the_new_science_of_forgiveness
4. http://stress.about.com/od/relationships/a/forgiveness.htm
5. http://stress.about.com/b/2008/02/28/todays-challenge-play-the-optimism-game.htm
6. Psalm 73:21
7. Leviticus 19:18
8. Matthew 6:14

Love

What's love got to do with it?

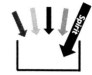

The English language uses one word to express the many facets of this concept. "I love dogs." "I love to sail." "I love you." We use this word in so many contexts, but it has such varied meanings. Ancient Greek contained several distinct words to refer to different types of love. While there is some overlap in their use and meaning, here is a general overview of five different Greek words for love:

- *Philia* →this word for love refers to a general type of love in the sense of friendship or affection. It includes the concept of loyalty to friends, family and community.

- *Éros* →this denotes passionate love, including physical, sensual love. It does not just describe sexual love though; it includes emotional love and the feeling of love.

- *Agápe* →this Greek word refers to a general affection or a deeper love (i.e. "true love") than that of *éros*. Christians understand this type of love as the selfless, sacrificial and unconditional love displayed by God in Jesus Christ.

- *Storge* →this word for love was used by the ancient Greeks to denote natural love, as in that of familial relationships. It is almost solely used to describe the love between a parent and child or brother and sister.

- *Mania*→is not really love in a positive sense at all. It is more the idea of "lust" or "obsession". It is the intense desire to possess something or someone (e.g. kleptomania).

Love is a complicated topic, pondered by the ancient Greeks, idolized by songwriters and examined by modern science. According to psychologist Abraham Maslow, the need to belong and be loved is one of the five basic motivations of human beings. He theorized that, next to the fulfillment of our human needs for food, water and safety/security, our need for love and belonging motivates us to create social networks of community in order to fulfill these needs. Maslow suggested that an individual's level of happiness correlated directly with the level of fulfillment of each of these five basic needs. A study done to test Maslow's conclusions in 2011 indicated that even in situations where fundamental physiological needs were not completely fulfilled (e.g. food, water, shelter, etc.), individuals could still report happiness due to feeling loved in their social relationships.

Research, on the topic of romantic love, shows that it takes between 90 seconds and 4 minutes to decide if you are attracted to someone. That attraction is based 7% on what is actually said, 55% on body language and 38% on the tone and speed of voice. Helen Fisher of Rutgers University has proposed three stages of love: lust, attraction and attachment. Fisher studied the hormones released in the early days of romantic relationships and discovered patterns in the neurotransmitters that were released in couples' brains at different points in their relationships. In stage one, she noted that testosterone and estrogen were the dominating hormones affecting the brains of men and women respectively. In the attraction stage, Fisher noted the increased presence of adrenaline, dopamine and serotonin in couples' brains. These neurotransmitters are responsible for symptoms such as a racing heart, increased energy, a decreased need for sleep and constant thoughts of the object of one's attraction. Finally, in stage three, Fisher noticed increased levels of the hormone oxytocin. Oxytocin is a neurotransmitter released during orgasm. Research suggests that the more sex a couple has, the stronger their bond will become.

Helen Fisher proposed that these chemicals released over the course of romantic relationships were nature's way of ensuring reproduction. Investigations conducted on the brain activity of individuals experiencing passionate love, as opposed to maternal or unconditional love, suggests that the physiological effects experienced by those "in love" can augment cognitive function.

Oxytocin is the same hormone released in women after childbirth. It cements the bond between a mother and baby. A mother's love is a powerful force. A study recently conducted at the Washington University School of Medicine investigated the effect of a mother's love on the physiology of her child. Brain images were taken of children from both nurturing and non-nurturing home environments. The children from nurturing home environments had hippocampal volumes 10% greater than children from less nurturing environments. The hippocampus is the region of the brain important for learning, memory and stress responses. Additional supporting research has confirmed the positive impact a nurturing home environment has on a child's ability to learn in school.

We can see that love has a significant impact on our quality of life from a scientific perspective. So what does that look like? If we say we are loved, what does that mean in day-to-day life? Dr. Gary Chapman, pastor, marriage counselor and author, has written a book called The Five Love Languages. This book came as the result of years of marriage counseling and the observation of patterns Dr. Chapman noticed in his clients over time. He discovered that spouses often came to counseling with complaints that fit into five different categories. "You do not spend any time with me." "You did not bring me anything from your business trip." "You never do anything around the house." "If I did not initiate, you would never touch me." "All you ever do is criticize me." Dr. Chapman concluded that humans receive love in five different ways: quality time, the giving of gifts, acts of service, physical touch and words of affirmation. His book explains each of these "love languages" and provides an inventory to help individuals discover their love languages. Do you know what yours is? (please refer to the following link for The Five Love Language Quiz http://www.iacac.org/wp-content/uploads/2012/05/D31-I-Hate-Your-Job-The-5-Love-Languages.pdf)

Once you are aware of what your love language is, it is important to communicate that knowledge to those closest to you. Dr. Chapman uses the imagery of a "love tank" in his book to describe how loved we feel at any given time. When those around us are communicating love in a way that we understand, our love tank will be full. If our communication lines are crossed, we may feel unloved, even though others are trying to love us. At NaturoMedic.com, we recognize the importance of maintaining a full love tank for one's overall health. Whether this love comes from the relationship of a husband and wife, a mother and daughter, or close friends, we encourage you to invest in what will last forever.

"Three things will last forever – faith, hope, and love – and the greatest of these is love"

References:
1. http://www.thecanadianencyclopedia.com/articles/inuit-words-for-snow-and-ice
2. http://en.wikipedia.org/wiki/Greek_words_for_love
3. http://chrismlegg.com/2009/10/01/5-greek-words-for-love-agape/
4. http://chrismlegg.com/2009/10/01/5-greek-words-for-love-agape/
5. http://psychology.about.com/od/theoriesofpersonality/a/hierarchyneeds.htm
6. http://psychology.about.com/b/2011/07/05/putting-maslows-hierarchy-of-needs-to-the-test.htm
7. http://www.youramazingbrain.org/lovesex/sciencelove.htm
8. http://www.livescience.com/18196-maternal-support-child-brain.html
9. http://www.5lovelanguages.com/faqs/love-languages/
10. http://www.iacac.org/wp-content/uploads/2012/05/D31-I-Hate-Your-Job-The-5-Love-Languages.pdf
11. 1 Corinthians 13:13

Spiritual Doors

Caveat Emptor: Let the Buyer Beware

Some may think it strange to find a section on spiritual doors in a book about health. We at NaturoMedic.com would tend to disagree. The growing fascination we observe in society and Hollywood with "other-worldly" creatures and fantasies leads us to believe this section is increasingly more relevant for our readers than it would have been twenty, or even ten, years ago. The number of books, movies and television shows produced in recent years about supernatural phenomena and the secret battle between good and evil, light and dark, give us reason to share some perspective on this spiritual factor of health. Belief systems encompassing a menagerie of spiritual and religious traditions including Gaia philosophy, astrology, Wicca, holistic health, Buddhism, Taoism, and the Native American cultures, to name a few, can open up spiritual doors. Casting spells, accessing animal spirits, placing curses, accessing spirit guides, or "channeling", practicing blood bonds, watching horror films, using Ouija boards or repeatedly visiting haunted houses can make us vulnerable to unwanted consequences. In the same way that we understand various environmental and physical factors to be influencers of health, we at NaturoMedic.com recognize that spiritual factors come into play as well.

Anyone receiving and acting on advice from a channeller or "enlightened being" is possibly giving up their free will to that entity and allowing it to get a foot in the door of their mind. The existence of demonic entities and oppression is real but there are very few who can and will address this issue when it does come up. Before going further and relying on that guidance, check their resume (is that possible?), references and ask questions. We at NaturoMedic.com desire to give a warning to those involved in various enlightenment streams: **caveat emptor** or "let the buyer beware." Medical Doctor W. Brugh Joy, who became an eastern guru, stated: "Not one person knows what [psychic power] is or all of its aspects and no one has ever known, despite attempts over thousands of years to master this knowledge. Tapping these energies is fire and the consequences…can be psychosis, aggravation of neuroses, acceleration of disease processes and suicide." Jacob Needleman, a professor at the University of California at Berkeley has said: "[In the psychic market], there's no Better Business Bureau. Let the Buyer Beware. You should be open minded, but not so open minded that your brains fall out."

"People who dabble in this area may start out as feeling in control of the spirits they are accessing, but will they continue to be in control or will they become a pawn in a much bigger chess game? A chess game in which they have no concept of the rules or the end results of the game." At NaturoMedic.com, we feel it is important to educate oneself about the implications of our choices and actions in every area of life. Should you wish to read more on this topic, please refer to www.NaturoMedic.com.

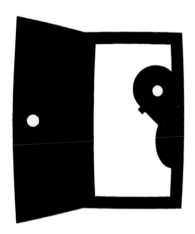

References:
1. W. Brugh Joy MD, Joy's Way (Thatcher, 1979) pg. 8-9.
2. US News and World Report p 69.
3. Michael A Prytula ND, Staff Meeting May 2004.

Part II: Your Road Map to Success

Chapter 8

Recommended Initiatives

*must be a patient of NaturoMedic.com in order to receive treatment protocol

Changing Habits

From early childhood, human beings are conditioned by our parents, our culture and our environment to do things a certain way. Our worldview is shaped by the things we are told we can and cannot do. As we reach adulthood, we are free to continue in the things we learned as children or to reevaluate life and make our own choices. All of these influences lead to the creation of the habits that make up who we are. It is precisely because habits are so automatic that we rarely stop to think about the enormous role they play in shaping our behavior, and in fact our lives (Shawn Achor).

We all have habits – some good, some bad. Or are they? Ask the alcoholic acting under the influence of alcohol if drinking alcohol is a "good" habit? Ask the emotional eater in the middle of a binge if this is a "good" habit? Ask the marijuana smoker while he is getting high if smoking marijuana is a "good" habit? No doubt the answers you receive will seek to justify each behavior. If it feels good, it must be good. Right?

At NaturoMedic.com we have decided to change our vocabulary with respect to habits. We prefer to think of these patterns of behavior as successful or unsuccessful habits. Ask the alcoholic, marijuana smoker, emotional eater or sugar junkie if they have an unsuccessful habit. They will most likely agree. Maybe you are struggling with your own unsuccessful habit? Perhaps a specific habit is making you late for work or causing behavior changes that you do not like? Now the motivation for changing your unsuccessful habit becomes greater success: with work, in relationships, etc. We all want success in some form, do we not?

So how does one go about changing unsuccessful habits? First, it is important to remember that it takes 21 days to make a habit. The **21-day** habit encourages an individual to focus on establishing one successful habit over the course of 21 days. One has only so much will power to exert, so it is important to conquer one item at a time. We have seen success when using this method to change habits, but we have noticed that other tools may be needed for it to be truly successful.

A study by Gail Matthews from Dominican University revealed some interesting conclusions about the benefits of setting goals. Matthews assigned volunteers from a broad range of ages and backgrounds to five different groups. Each group was asked to determine goals for a four-week time period; some were to just think about them; some were to write their goals down, and others were asked to write progress reports to a friend as they completed their goals. The group that was asked to write down their goals had 50% more success in completing them than those who were only asked to think about their goals. The group that was asked to be accountable to a friend for completing their goals saw the highest level of success by fulfilling 76% of their stated goals. These conclusions suggest that writing out goals and being accountable to keep them is a great way to achieve the things we want to do. Take Alcoholics Anonymous, for example; accountability is a huge part of their success, requiring each participant to have a sponsor. For goal-setting to be effective, summary feedback that reveals progress is a key component to your strategy.

One other helpful tool for creating successful habits is the **20-second rule**. The 20-second rule is a psychological construct based upon happiness research popularized by Shawn Achor in his book The Happiness Advantage. The 20-second rule comes from the concept of activation energy. How long does it take the average person to initiate something? Research suggests that people are far more likely to do things if it takes 20 seconds or less to initiate the activity. If the activation time takes greater than 20 seconds, they most likely will not do it. In Achor's book, a research study was cited in which ice cream consumption in a cafeteria was cut in half by simply closing the lid of the ice cream cooler.

This concept can be a powerful tool in eliminating unsuccessful habits. After reading about this concept, one of NaturoMedic.com's practitioners put it to the test on David, a man of the cloth who had a smoking habit. We discovered that David only smoked in his car. He would get in the car to travel somewhere and automatically reach for a cigarette. After explaining the 20-second rule to David, we agreed that he should try keeping his cigarettes in the trunk and remove all lighters from the vehicle. This required David to pull over, retrieve his cigarettes, find a lighter, and get back on the road every time he wanted to smoke. No one can do that in less than 20 seconds! David has now almost completely removed his unsuccessful habit of smoking from his life.

This tool can be applied to all kinds of unsuccessful habits. If you are an email addict, bury your email folder in 20 other folders to increase the time it takes you to open it. For those who eat when stress levels rise, empty your cupboards of sweets and chips.

The 20-second rule can also be used to create successful habits. Another patient, Matt, was a long-term drinker who needed to make a change. While driving under the influence of alcohol, he was stopped by a NY state trooper just outside his residence and mercifully released without severe consequences. He needed to find help. We determined that he most often drank at a local pub on his way home from work. Matt also revealed that his drinking was getting in the way of his social time for golf. Taking into account the 20-second rule, we agreed that Matt should program his GPS to take him home from work a different way – right past his favourite golf course. He began keeping his golf clubs in the trunk so that he always had the equipment to golf at any time. These minor changes led to a reduction in Matt's alcohol consumption by 80%! Not only that, but he was able to replace an unsuccessful habit with a life-giving successful habit.

It is important to remember that human **willpower** is actually very limited. In The Happiness Advantage, Achor points out that the more we are required to use our willpower, the more worn-out it gets. A willpower study documented in Achor's book gave an example of this fact. Three groups of college students were asked to refrain from eating three hours before an experiment. When the groups arrived at the lab, they were each given different instructions regarding two plates of food. One plate contained chocolate cookies, the other radishes. The first group was told they could have as many radishes as they wanted, but no cookies. The second group was allowed to eat off of either plate. The third group was given no food at all. After being required to follow these instructions for a certain period of time, each group was given a set of geometric puzzles to solve. Which group gave up on solving the puzzles first? Group One. It appears that this group had used up all of their willpower in resisting the chocolate chip cookies and had little mental energy left over to persevere in solving the puzzles.

This limitation of willpower is what makes habits so powerful. Once an activity has become routine/normal (i.e. a habit), we no longer need mental energy to make it happen; we do it automatically much like riding a bike or driving. This frees us up to focus on the next thing. This is why the 21-day rule and the 20-second concept are such valuable tools in one's health journey. As we develop healthier habits in place of our unsuccessful ones, we will eventually find ourselves living the lives we want, one habit at a time.

These principles of incremental change and habit development can easily be applied to every area of one's life. In his book The Likeability Factor, Tim Sanders talks about four habits of character that will cause you to be more likeable: friendliness, relevance, empathy and realness. Sanders postulates that the more you are liked, the happier your life will be. While that philosophy gives others far too much control over one's happiness for our liking, we do recognize the importance of intentionally developing character. If you find yourself lacking in courage, integrity, positivity, kindness, temperance or gratitude, evaluate your habits and begin making small steps in the direction you want to go.

Another area where these principles may be useful is with respect to gaining authority. We all want authority in some way. We want the right to choose how to live our lives, to choose where we live, what we do, who we spend time with. Authority can be achieved in two ways. We can pursue it or we can have it granted to us. To pursue authority means to take authority because of our title. This kind of authority comes with accountability and responsibility, both of which are usually unwanted. For example, teenagers want the authority to drive, a common rite of passage in North America. What they soon learn is that, in order to sustain this authority, they must be responsible to the rules of the road and give account to the law keepers should they fail to obey. Unfortunately, much of society pursues authority in this manner. Governments, politicians, lawyers and bureaucrats want authority, but rarely do they want the accountability and responsibility that come with it. Doctors want authority over your body, but they do not want to be held responsible for the consequences of poor decisions. At NaturoMedic.com, we feel authority should follow the demonstration of willingness for accountability and responsibility. This is another arena in which the development of healthy character habits (e.g. integrity) could be of benefit on numerous levels.

To summarize, incremental changes can bring about significant results when we are working toward a larger goal. So while the obstacles to health transformation may seem at times insurmountable, there is hope when we take it one day at a time. Start small. Get rid of unsuccessful habits. Pursue successful habits. Take responsibility for where you are in life now. Be accountable to yourself and those around you. Stick to a plan that works.

…Remember

Changing Habits: The Rule of 21™.

- Will power is finite

- Only change 1 habit every 21 days

- To establish a successful habit it must take less than 21 seconds (20 seconds) to initiate it

- To break oneself of an unsuccessful habit it must take over 21 seconds (20 seconds) to initiate it

- Write it down (50% success)

- Have a friend or your health care provider hold you accountable (76% success)

References:
1. http://michaelhyatt.com/life-plan
2. http://michaelhyatt.com/the-power-of-incremental-change-over-time.html
3. Achor, Shawn; The Happiness Advantage, 2010. Pgs. 145-170.
4. Sanders, Tim. The Likeability Factor.

Air Filters

With all the potential adverse health effects from the quality of air in the home it is natural to want to protect yourself and your family from the chemicals being released into the air (off-gassing). Filtering the air we breathe is one of the best ways to remove harmful agents. There are so many types of filters on the market today; knowing which one to buy can be confusing. It is important to do your research and purchase a good quality filter.

Up to 95% of the particles found in the air are small and not visible. When selecting a filter, look for the percentage capture (e.g. 95% or more) of total number respirable particles. Respirable particles are 10 microns in size or less (smaller than the thickness of a human hair). A typical furnace has a one inch thick rough filter which can remove most of the large particles. Pleated filters and mesh electrostatic filters are available for the furnace to help improve efficiency but are not very effective at trapping small particles.

To remove small particles, a HEPA (high-efficiency particulate air filter) or an electronic filter can be installed on your furnace. A HEPA filter can remove up to 98% of the small particles including ones that are 0.3 microns in size. Electronic filters can remove even smaller particles but are not very effective at removing large particles. These filters may require weekly cleaning to maintain good performance as both filters can become quickly clogged with larger particles. A rough filter can be installed in front to prescreen out the big particles. Please note that washing and vacuuming filters will expose you to concentrated contaminants. Cleaning the filter outdoors and with a mask can help protect your lungs. It is important to note that filtration tends to work best the closer it is to the person. Many people do not permanently live in their basements by the furnace so portable room filters might be considered as they are more effective.

The ability of filters to remove odours is often a concern. Carbon and some chemisorbent filters can remove gas molecules including formaldehyde and other volatile organic compounds. Carbon filters are best compared by weight. The heavier the filter the more gas molecules (odours) it will remove.

Ultraviolet light (UV) generators are advertised as a method for purifying the air in your home. These are not filters, nor are they a substitute for a good filter. These units can kill bacteria and viruses but their low efficiency filters are mainly to keep dust off of the UV bulb. Ozone generators have been shown to be beneficial in combatting mold, but these are also not air filters.

Below is a more detailed description of the potential filter types available for the home constructed by PuraHome, Air and Water Purification Specialists. A chart for comparative analysis has also been included.

(http://www.purahome.com/ 40 Secord Drive, Toll Free: 1-866-670-PURA
(7872) Telephone: 905-934-3168)

Plasmawave

Plasma is a charged gas. An alternating electrical discharge creates positive hydrogen ions and negative oxygen ions. These Plasma Ions known as PlasmaWave shoot into the air. They naturally seek out and surround allergens such as dust mites, bacteria, viruses and spores. When the PlasmaWave combines with water in the air, hydroxyls are created. Hydroxyls have been studied extensively all over the world including NASA and the US Army. Hydroxyls will surround the allergens and rob them of hydrogens in order to reform water. This renders the allergen inactive as shown by protein structure testing. The plasma also has the ability to reduce many airborne organic pollutants in the air in to simpler nontoxic substances such as carbon dioxide and water. These systems are usually portable and can be moved from room to room.

Ozone Systems

Ozone is a strong oxidizer. Ozone is unstable and thereby easily gives an oxygen atom to alter the chemical composition of gases by oxidizing them. It has little or no effect on solid particles although it may halt the growth of mold and bacteria and purify areas of toxins by oxidating them much like oxidized steel (rust), when used in high concentrations. Ozone is often referred to as "energized oxygen" or "pure air" suggesting that ozone is a healthy kind of oxygen. The truth is that Ozone is a toxic gas with vastly different chemical and toxicological properties from oxygen. Ozone can be harmful to and irritate the respiratory system. It is also the primary component of smog. Both the United States Environmental Protection Agency and Health Canada DO NOT APPROVE GENERATORS FOR USE IN OCCUPIED SPACE. (*N/A for medical ozone applications*)

UV Lights

Ultra Violet lights (germicidal lamps) or UV systems come in both a hot (8,000 hours life) and cold plasma (rate 36,000 hours life) lamp system. They produce a specific wavelength that has the ability to affect microbiological contaminants like mold and bacteria and to keep it from replicating. UV has no effect on solid particles and it does NOT remove anything from the air stream. UV lights are normally placed in the return air stream. It is important to understand that the speed of the air passing by the lights can minimize the effectiveness of the UV lights. Placing a UV light at or near the cooling coils may work better as the light can irradiate this moist area all the time and help in minimizing the growth of mold or bacteria in the coils. Some UV lights have an additional wavelength that can split oxygen to create short-term ozone that will help sanitize the coils more efficiently as well as reduce spores and odours. If designed properly, the ozone will have dissipated quickly in the cold air return. UV lights are an ancillary piece of equipment and should always be used in conjunction with an air filtration system

Ion Generators

These devices produce negative ions that charge the particles in the air. The charged particles then attach themselves to both a positive and neutral surface area. This could be a wall, floor, furniture, ceiling, etc. Once the particles lose their charge, they will become airborne again.

There are many options available and many items to consider when selecting an air filter. Make sure to be well informed prior to making a purchase in order to protect your home efficiently. In addition to getting an air filter, there are some steps you can do as well. Open the windows in new homes and new cars for a few days to allow the formaldehyde and VOCs to be off gassed into the air. Bring greenery into the home, especially plants that help purify the formaldehyde specifically (e.g. Rubber plants). Through the soil, greenery can be a source of mold. By covering the soil with tin foil this problem can be reduced. Purifying the air we breathe can help reduce respiratory problems, asthma, allergies and long-term adverse effects.

References:
1. http://www.calgaryallergy.ca/Articles/English/Adobe/Air%20Filter%20Re view.pdf
2. http://www.purahome.com/articles/files/Air_Cleaning_Technology_Comp arison-_alternate_systems.pdf
3. http://www.air-purifier.org/comparisons.html
4. http://webecoist.com/2009/04/08/air-purifying-plants/

Air Cleaning Method Effectiveness Comparison

0 = no effect 1 = little effect 2 = some effect 3 = medium effect 4 = strong effect 5 = most effective

Contaminant	Plasma Wave	HEPA Filters	Electronic Filters	Carbon Filters	Negative Ionizers (Ionic)	Standard UV Germicidal Light (CAUTION EYES)	Corona Discharge Ozone Generators (EXTREME DANGER)
Airborne Bacteria	5	3	2	1	1	4	5
Surface Bacteria	5	0	0	0	0	0	5
Airborne Viruses	5	1	1	0	1	4	5
Surface Viruses	5	0	0	0	0	0	5
Airborne Particulates	3	3	3	1	3	0	1
Gases	5	0	0	0	0	2	4
Odors	5	0	0	3	0	0	5
Destroys Contaminants	5	0	2	0	0	3	5
Coverage Area	5	2	2	2	2	2	5

Environmental Allergies

There are thousands of different types of particulates present in the air throughout the year that can lead to allergy symptoms. Knowing when these counts are elevated may help to prepare you for days that will create the most symptoms and may also help reduce your exposure. The weather network offers daily pollen forecast available during allergy season. Take a look at http://www.theweathernetwork.com/pollenfx/canpollen_en to see the seasonal variation for your area. The symptoms you often experience with an allergy resemble a cold. It can be difficult to tell whether the sneezing and the itchy, watery eyes are from an allergy or a sickness (cold or flu). The first step is to distinguish between these two possibilities. There are a few ways in which you can do this:

1. Most vehicles made since 2005 have a HEPA filter (High efficiency particulate air filter). Typically one would push the recycle air button in the cabin to engage it. Once engaged, breathe the filtered air. If you notice that your symptoms improve drastically within 5 minutes, you can assume it is the substances in the air that is causing your symptoms. Removing these particles from your environment can help reduce your allergy symptoms (*please refer to Air Filters for more information*).

2. Visit a lake on days when there is an onshore breeze (wind coming off the lake onto the shore with no land for one mile). The onshore breeze has no pollen or mold spores so you will naturally clear up as the allergen particles slowly dissipate from your nasal passageways. If your symptoms improve, you know you are not suffering from a cold. It also might be good to have fun by the lake or on the water and be allergy free.

Treatment:

1. Sanctuary: Make your bedroom an allergy free sanctuary. If you are being disturbed all night by allergies, you are not going to be well rested or refreshed in the morning. Keep any clothing or items exposed to potential allergens out of the room. Keep animals out of your room, especially animals that are also outdoors. Close your window and run the fan on the furnace (fitted with an efficient air filter).

2. Shower: Taking a shower before bed will remove any allergen spores embedded on the skin, nose and in the hair (you must use shampoo). This will help to keep your pillow free from substances that can trigger symptoms. If you sleep close to your loved one, they might need to shower too.

3. Purchase a HEPA filter to operate in your bedroom (*please refer to Air filters for more recommendations*).

4. Supplementation: These suggestions will be individualized according to the recommendations of your NaturoMedic.com Naturopathic Doctor.

Exercise

Exercise, as discussed in the lifestyle section, increases circulation, muscle strength, longevity, mood, etc. The health benefits of exercise are dependent upon the frequency, intensity and duration of the exercise, not to mention the type of activity. Before entering a workout program, make sure you use an appropriate amount of intensity to reach your desired effect.

Cardiovascular Fitness

Aerobic activity is one of the best methods for improving the ability of the heart, lungs and blood vessels to function at an optimal level during exercise and at rest. This form of activity helps with the delivery of oxygen to tissue, thus ensuring that energy demands are being met. Continuous, rhythmic activity performed at an appropriate intensity in order to increase cardiac output is an essential criterion for aerobic exercise (ex. cycling, running, cross-country skiing, skating, hiking, etc.).

Tips to Improve Cardio Conditioning:

1. **Know your Intensity**: calculate your maximum heart rate (MHR) to know which range will apply the appropriate amount of strenuous exercise. This range should be between 60%-90% of your MHR, also referred to as comfortable-hard. Subtract your age from 220 and then multiply this figure by 0.60 and 0.90 to yield your target heart rate. Ex. 220-35=185 beats per min (bpm), 185 x 0.6= 111 & 185 x 0.9=166.5. Your target is between 111bpm- 166bpm.

2. **Duration**: Warm-up and cool-down should each be from 5-10 min.
   - children ages 5 to 11 and youth ages 12 to 17 should:
     a. accumulate at least 60 minutes of moderate to vigorous intensity physical activity daily
     b. include vigorous-intensity activities at least 3 days per week.
   - adults aged 18 to 64 should:
     a. accumulate at least 150 minutes of moderate to vigorous intensity aerobic physical activity per week, in 10 minutes bouts or more.

3. **Frequency**: daily sessions are recommended. *Note: if first starting out it is important to take a day off to allow the body to rest and recuperate. Work up towards the appropriate intensity, duration and frequency. Always check in with yourself.*

Muscular Fitness

Anaerobic activity includes effective exercises that use resistance to build muscle and bone. Anaerobic exercise does not use oxygen for energy and therefore is not done for long periods at a time. Lactic acid is produced as a by-product which can affect muscle action and function. These types of exercises use muscles at high intensity for short periods of time. Muscular strength and endurance are two important aspects of any exercise program. These help strengthen the body for the requirements of daily life and prevent the loss of lean body tissue that often occurs with age.

Tips to Improve Muscular Conditioning
1. **Intensity**: the weight should be enough to be able to perform 5 to 15 repetitions. You would like the muscle to feel a little tired or to burn toward the end of your reps.
2. **Duration**: one to three sets of 5 to 15 repetitions are often performed. Always rest for at least one minute between sets.
3. **Frequency**: 3 to 5 days a week. Remember to always allow a muscle group to rest for one day before returning to that program (e.g. Monday -lower body workout. Tuesday- upper body workout)
4. Children complete activities to strengthen muscle and bone at least three days per week.

When beginning a new exercise program, you may find that you are not able to complete all of the exercises as often or for the desired length of time as you would like. It is important to begin slowly and progress up to your fitness goals. Doing too much too fast can lead to injury, pain and the abandonment of your exercise program. Take your time and enjoy the endorphin energy boost. Remember to stretch after your workout. This step is quite often skipped over, but it is necessary to maintain proper range of motion in your joints. Finally, please do not forget to breathe throughout both the cardiovascular and muscular conditioning portions. Breathing is not only essential to life, but it also helps with the detoxification process.

References:
1. Pizzorno & Murray. Textbook of Natural Medicine. 3rd ed. Vol. I. Churchill Livingstone. 2006.
2. http://www.cbc.ca/news/health/story/2011/01/24/fitness-guidelines.html

Water Filters

Clean drinking water is important for maintaining optimal health for both you and your family. The need for water filtering systems is a growing concern for many. In 1993, over 100 people died from *cryptosporidium* contaminated water in Milwaukee, Wisconsin. Seven deaths from *E. coli* tainted water occurred in Walkerton, Ontario in 2000. Our tap water is regularly affected by acid rain, pesticides, heavy metals and toxic waste, all of which can be very dangerous to your health. Filtering and purifying our water supply has become a priority to many. There are many water filters available on the market today. Whether it is a home system for the faucet, refrigerator or shower, it is important to be familiar with the product you are purchasing. Understanding what the filtering system is capable of prior to making a purchase is very important. One major benefit regarding water filters is that the vast majority have to follow strict guidelines. The Environmental Protection Agency and Health Canada monitor this industry far more closely than the bottled water industry. In fact, there are no federal filtration or disinfection requirements in place for bottled water companies.

When water passes through a water filter, a filter media absorbs and screens for particles. There are a wide range of water filters, purifiers and methods of water purification available on the market today. There is no single filter or treatment that will eliminate 100% of every contaminant from your water. Many technologies target only a specific type of contaminant and may be completely ineffective against others. **Important factors to consider when selecting your system are: does your filter conserve water and energy? Does it eliminate heavy metals, chemicals and microorganisms? How much maintenance does it require? How often do you have to replace the filter? How easy is it to move (are you a tenant?)? Do you want whole house or localized filtration (drinking water)? What is the cost?** For the most popular water filtration methods and drinking water brands on the market refer to the water filter comparison charts at www.naturomedic.com. The charts compare the performance of carbon, ceramic, reverse osmosis and distilled filtration systems. They also demonstrate how the quality of water changes over time for distillation, reverse osmosis and carbon filters.

There is no filter on the market capable of removing 100 percent of all contaminants. Do your research and select the system that is best for you and your family. **Remember if you do not have a water filter, you are the filter!**

For additional information on water filters please visit: http://www.purahome.com/articles/files/water_cleaning_technology_comparis on-contaminant_removal.pdf

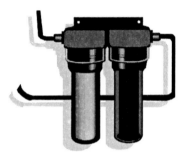

References:
1. http://www.guide2waterfilters.com/water-filter-types/drinking-water-systems.aspx
2. http://www.aquatechnology.net/system_comparisons.html
3. http://www.nrdc.org/water/drinking/bw/exesum.asp

Chapter 9

Optimizing Interventions

*must be a patient of NaturoMedic.com in order to receive treatment protocol

Detoxification

Detoxification is an important elimination process the body uses daily to remove toxins and prevent their accumulation in the body. It does not matter how many good things you put into your body if you cannot take out the garbage. Your body is the house of your soul. If you accumulate garbage in one room of your house that will attract flies (microorganisms, abnormal cells, cancerous cells...). Antibiotics, antivirals, chemotherapy and radiation kill the flies (bacteria, viruses and cancer cells), but if you do not do anything to get rid of the garbage, the flies will come back.

The liver, intestines and kidneys are the primary organs responsible for this, however there are actually 5 methods of detoxification employed by the body. **Toxins that are not removed are stored in fat tissue and bone.**

Organ	Method	Toxin Solubility
Skin	Excretion through sweat	Fat & Water
Liver	**Filtering of the blood, bile secretion, phase I detoxification, phase II detoxification**	**Fat**
Intestines	Mucosal detoxification, excretion through feces	Mostly Fat Some Water
Kidneys	Excretion through urine	Water
Lungs	Excretion through respiration	Water

Generally, we have two types of toxins: water soluble and fat soluble. Water soluble toxins can be dissolved in water, whereas fat soluble toxins are dissolved in fat. The liver plays the most crucial role in fat soluble detoxification. It filters blood to remove large toxins, synthesizes and secretes bile to remove fat soluble toxins and disassembles unwanted chemicals with enzymes. This disassembly process requires two steps. Phase I will directly neutralize a toxin or will modify the chemical into a form that can be neutralized by Phase II. The liver detoxifies almost 2 liters of blood every minute and 99% of bacteria and toxins. However, when the liver is damaged, the amount of toxins that remain in the blood increases by 10 times.

Phase I Detoxification

Phase I utilizes a group of enzymes known as cytochrome P450. There are roughly 50-100 enzymes in this system that either directly neutralize some chemicals or convert them into forms to be eliminated by Phase II enzymes. The activity of cytochrome P450 enzymes varies individually based on genetics, exposure level to chemical toxins and nutritional status. The variation in activity is responsible for the variation in risk for disease. For example, there are differences in smokers' abilities to detoxify carcinogens. Some people can smoke and only sustain modest lung damage while others develop cancer. In addition those with underactive Phase I detoxification will experience intolerances to multiple substances, including caffeine and perfumes.

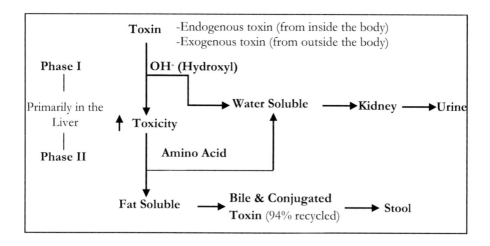

Cytochrome P450 metabolizes a chemical to a less toxic form, making it water soluble or converting it to a more chemically active form. This more active form must be quickly removed from the body by Phase II to prevent a potential problem. Therefore the rate at which Phase I produces activated metabolites must be balanced by the rate at which Phase II processes them. An imbalance between the two phases can occur when a person is exposed to large amounts of toxins or for long periods of time. The critical nutrients become depleted allowing for the highly active forms from Phase I to accumulate. The activity of Phase I enzymes can also decrease with age, lack of physical activity and reduced circulation. Copper, magnesium, zinc and vitamin C are vital nutrients required by Phase I enzymes.

The following chart demonstrates substances detoxified by Phase I as well as drugs that inhibit Phase I enzymes.

Chemicals Detoxified by Phase I			
Drug:	Over the counter:	Food:	Environmental:
Phenytoin	Acetaminophen	Caffeine	Alcohol
Codeine	Ibuprofen	Vanilla	Insecticides
Erythromycin	Salicylates		CCl_4
Warfarin			Cigarette smoke
Amitryptyline			Charcoal-broiled
Prednisone			meat
Phenobarbital			
Steroids			
Inhibitors of Phase I			
Drugs:			
Benzodiazepines	Stomach acid secretion blocking drugs		
Antihistamines	Antifungals (ketoconazole etc…)		

Phase II Detoxification

In Phase II, various liver enzymes attach small chemicals to the toxin, a process known as conjugation. This reaction either neutralizes a toxin or makes it more easily excreted by the kidneys or bowels. There are seven pathways of detoxification in Phase II, each requiring certain nutrients and energy to function properly.

The following chart describes the seven Phase II pathways and provides information on the nutrients needed for each step and the substances that can decrease its activity.

Phase II System	Nutrients	Inhibitors	Detoxifies	Dysfunction Indicator	Other
Glutathione conjugation	-Glutathione (cysteine (a.a), glutamic acid (a.a) and glycine (a.a)) -B$_6$ -NAC -Protein (whey)	-Selenium deficiency -Vitamin B$_2$ deficiency -Glutathione deficiency -Zinc deficiency	-Acetaminophen -Nicotine -Organo-phosphates (pesticide, herbicide)	-Chronic exposure to chemical toxins -Chronic alcohol consumption	-Elimination of fat soluble compounds, especially heavy metals like mercury and lead is dependent upon adequate levels of glutathioine -Vitamin C, N-acetylcysteine (NAC), glycine and methionine will help increase
Amino acid conjugation	-Glycine (a.a) -Taurine (a.a) -Glutamine (a.a) -Arginine (a.a) -Protein (whey)	-Low protein	-Benzoate -Aspirin	Intestinal toxicity, toxemia of pregnancy	
Methylation	-S-adenosyl-methionine -Protein (whey)	-Folic acid -Vitamin B$_{12}$ deficiency	-Dopamine -Epinephrine -Histamine -Thiouracil	-Premenstrual syndrome -Estrogen excess -Cholestasis	-Methylation involves conjugating methyl groups to toxins -Most of the methyl groups used for detoxification come from S-adenosylmethionine (SAMe) -SAMe is synthesized from the amino acid methionine, which requires vitamin B$_{12}$ and folic acid

191

Phase II System	Nutrients	Inhibitors	Detoxifies	Dysfunction Indicator	Other
Sulfation	-Cysteine (a.a) -Methionine (a.a) -Molybdenum -Protein (whey)	-NSAIDS (i.e.: aspirin) -Food dyes -Molybdenum deficiency	-Dyes -Coumarin -Acetaminophen -Estrogen -Testosterone -Thyroid hormones -Methyl-dopa	-Intestinal toxicity -Parkinson's disease -Alzheimer's disease -Rheumatoid arthritis	- Sulfation is the conjugation of toxins with sulfur-containing compounds - Sulfation is also a primary route for the elimination of neurotransmitters, dysfunction in this system may contribute to the development of some nervous system disorders
Acetylation	-Acetyl-CoA -Protein (whey)	-Vitamin B1, B5, C deficiency	-Sulfa drugs		Those with sensitivities/allergies to sulfa medication indicates poor acetylation - Dependent on B1, B5 and Vitamin C
Glucuronidation	- Glucuronic acid -Protein (whey)	- Non-steroidal anti-inflammatory drugs	- Acetaminophen -Morphine -Diazepam -Digitalis -Aspirin -Benzoates -Vanillin	-Gilbert's disease	

Phase II System	Nutrients	Inhibitors	Detoxifies	Dysfunction Indicator	Other
Sulfoxidation	- Molybdenum -Protein (whey)		- Sulfites, garlic compounds	- Adverse reactions to sulfite food additives, garlic -asthma reactions after eating foods with preservatives - strong urine odour after eating asparagus	- sulfur containing molecules in drugs and food (sulfite food additives) are metabolized and removed from the body

Protein

The metabolism of toxic chemicals and drugs is highly dependent upon protein and amino acid status in the body. Increased toxicity of chemical compounds and drugs has been connected with protein deficiency. Herbicide and fungicide accumulation have been shown to be increased several fold by low protein consumption. Low protein diets decrease cytochrome P450 activity, increase lead toxicity and increase the immune system's susceptibility to disease from pesticides. Protein is essential for proper functioning of all the Phase II detoxification pathways. Whey protein is one of the most important sources.

Bowel Excretion

Phase II requires the synthesis and secretion of bile. Each day the liver produces about 1 liter of bile which serves as a carrier for many toxic substances to be dumped into the intestines. These substances must be removed immediately to prevent their reabsorption into the system. Fiber, such as psyllium, absorbs the toxins carried by bile to the intestines and facilitates rapid excretion by the bowels. If bile elimination becomes inhibited, toxins can remain in the lives longer than desired.

Gallstones, "sludge", alcohol, thyroid conditions, constipation, oral contraceptives and other medications are just a few factors that can impair bile flow. Normal bowel action allows for 94% bile reabsorption. The fat soluble toxins excreted with it are recycled as part of the body's starvation prevention program. Constipation however would allow for 99% reabsorption. Fiber prevents liver recirculation and increases the amount of fecal bile acids by **400%.**

Systemic Detoxification

1. Avoidance: Reduce daily toxic burden (food, environment, etc.)

2. Supplementation: Help the body handle the toxic load (support detoxification pathways)

3. Cleansing/Detoxification: Remove of the toxic accumulation (fasting, saunas, colonics…)

Fasting

Fasting is one of the oldest known therapies that dates back over 3000 years. Fasting has been used in the treatment of: high blood pressure, obesity, chemical poisoning, rheumatoid arthritis, autoimmune disease, allergies, psoriasis, eczema, thrombophlebitis, leg ulcers, IBS, asthma and mood disorders. A professional organization involved in the study and promotion of fasting is the International Association of Hygienic Physicians (IAHP). It is composed of doctors specializing in therapeutic fasting as an integral part of total health care. One of the most significant studies regarding fasting and detoxification involved patients who had inadvertently ingested rice oil contaminated with polychlorinated-biphenyls (PCBs) in Taiwan. All patients reported improvement in symptoms and some observed "dramatic" relief, after undergoing 7-10 days of fasting. **The level of circulating chemicals in their blood increased due to the elevated rate of fat break down. Once the detoxification pathways caught up with the processing and elimination of fat soluble toxins, transformative changes occurred**. Thus the fat soluble PCBs were released from storage into the bloodstream at higher than normal rates. The liver's detoxification process is responsible for removing the substances through Phase I and Phase II *(please refer to Fasting for more information)*.

Saunas (48°C- 57°C)
Saunas stimulate one of the basic methods of detoxification by the body. **When the body sweats** toxins are released through the skin. One research article studied the exposure of 14 firemen to highly toxic PCBs using saunas. The firemen underwent 2-3 weeks of detoxification, through dieting and using saunas, after developing neuropsychological problems 6 months after a transformer fire explosion. Their memory was drastically improved following treatment. Saunas have multiple therapeutic benefits. They increase excretion of heavy metals (cadmium, lead), augment excretion of fat-soluble chemicals (PCBs) and accelerate fat breakdown throughout the body. Compounds become mobilized into the bloodstream through sweat. The compounds released can include cadmium, lead, mercury, nickel, bromide, chloride, chromium, copper, iron, potassium, sodium, magnesium, manganese and zinc.

Colonics
Colonic treatments clear compounds that have been dumped from the liver into the intestines. This therapeutic treatment further enhances the removal of bile and thus prevents their recirculation as 94% of toxins in the bile are recycled in Phase II. Colonics will also help with the absorption of water *(please refer to Colonics for more information)*.

Coffee Enemas
Coffee enemas have been a standard in detoxification protocols in the past, primarily due to triggering significant bile dumping and eliminating the reabsorption of toxins.

References:

1. Pizzorno, J. Textbook of Natural Medicine 3rd Ed. Elsevier. Churchill, Livingstone Page 347, 437-450.

2. Anticancer Res. 2000 Nov-Dec;20(6C):4785-92

3. Imamura M, Tung TC. A trial of fasting cure for PCB-poisoned patients in Taiwan. Am J Ind Med 1984;5:147-153.

4. Cohn JR, Emmett EA. The excretion of trace metals in human sweat. Ann Lin Lab Sci 1978; 8: 270-275

5. Schnare DW, Robinson PC. Reduction of the body burdens of hexachlorobenzene and polychlorinated biphenyls. IARC Sci Publ 1986;77: 597-603

6. Tretjak Z, Shields M, Beckmann SL. PCB reduction and clinical improvement by detoxification: an unexploited approach? Hum Exp Toxicol 1990; 9: 235-244

7. Lammintausta R, Syvalahti E, Pekkarnen A. Change in hormones reflecting sympathetic activity in Finnish sauna. Ann Clin Res 1976; 8: 266-271

Castor Oil Packs

The application of castor oil externally has been well explored throughout history. A castor oil pack can increase circulation, improve lymphatic function, decrease inflammation (internally and externally) and promote the elimination of toxins and the healing of tissues.

Materials Required:

- Undyed cotton towel or wool flannel of sufficient size to cover the abdomen

- A bottle of unrefined, cold pressed castor oil

- A hot water bottle or heating pad

- Fiber (Psyllium)

Directions:

1. Apply the castor oil over the abdomen (caution must be exercised; castor oil will stain clothes).

2. Place the towel or wool flannel over the area of the abdomen where the castor oil has been applied.

3. Apply a heating pad or hot water bottle, as warm as is comfortably bearable, on top of the towel or wool flannel. Apply a plastic water proof barrier between heating pad and castor oil towel.

4. Place another towel on top of the heating pad or hot water bottle.

5. Leave pack on for 20 minutes.

6. After the pack is completed, wash the oil off with warm water and baking soda (1 tsp. to 1 pint of warm water)

Cleansing Diet

The Cleansing Diet is designed for a 5-7-or 10-day period. The diet will provide you with all the nutrition you need while your body cleanses, detoxifies and heals. On this diet, calories are not counted nor are food weighed. **Strict attention** is given to the selection and quality of the food consumed during the diet. Below is a list of restricted and permitted foods.

"YES" FOODS	"NO" FOODS
Brown/wild/basmati rice	White rice
All vegetables (steamed, fresh, raw)	Sugar and sugar substitutes
Oatmeal, millet, amaranth, kamut, quinoa etc.	Citrus (except lemons)
	Candy of any kind (including gum)
All fruits (except citrus, lemon is OK)	Salt/sea salt, pepper
Lentils/peas/beans	Honey/maple syrup etc.
Hummus (chick peas pureed)	Fried food of any kind
Pure fruit juice sweetened cereals	Wheat noodles and wheat pastas
Brown rice cakes/noodles	including spelt
Nuts/seeds (raw, unsalted)	Coffee and tea including decaf
Soy/rice/almond/oat milks	Catfish
Fresh ocean going fish e.g. mackerel,	Shellfish i.e. lobster, clams, shrimp,
sardines, herring, snapper etc.	oysters, scallops
Tofu/tempeh (soybean products)	Wheat or wheat products
Pasture-fed/organic chicken, turkey,	Soya sauce
eggs	Commercial salad dressings
Dried, unsulphured fruits i.e. prunes,	Dairy/milk/cheese/sour cream
dates, figs, raisins etc.	Margarine/butter/soya margarine
Cold pressed/extra virgin oil (small	Breads (all kinds)
amounts only)	Vinegars
All herbs fresh/dried, non-salt herbal	French fries or chips (unless baked)
seasoning (Veg, nori/kelp etc.)	Alcoholic beverages
All natural seasonings/mixes	Red meats of any kind, beef or pork
Cayenne pepper/ginger/garlic	Seasonings with chemicals (i.e. MSG)
Herbal teas	
Potatoes boiled/baked	**Note:** Of course stay away from food
Hot air-popped popcorn	you know you are sensitive to!
Bean/seed sprouts	
Brown rice cereal, millet/rice flakes	
Seed/nut butters (tahini, tamari, etc.)	
Anything else that is not refined has no additives and is not on the **NO FOOD** list.	

The above chart may seem like a lot of restrictions. Some of the yes foods may be unfamiliar to you. For the duration of your Cleansing Diet as prescribed by your NaturoMedic.com ND, please refer to the **NaturoMedic™.com© Healthy Living Cookbook** located on our website **www.NaturoMedic.com** for recipes.

Please Note: Everything that is consumed while on the cleansing diet should not have any preservatives, no artificial colourings/flavourings, no stimulants, no salt, no pepper and no chemicals added what so ever. They should not be consumed from cans or plastic but glass containers. This cleansing diet is absolutely dairy and wheat free. All foods eaten during the diet should be unaltered by man as much as possible and fresh with all the wholesome goodness nature has made.

Guidelines:

a) Eat until you feel full but not engorged. It is better to eat six to eight small meals rather than three large ones daily. This will vary from person to person depending on your daily activities, demands and type of job.

b) Refrain from drinking 15-20 minutes before or after eating, even water. This dilutes the enzymes in the stomach needed to properly digest the foods eaten.

c) Eat all fruits and drink fruit juices separately from all other foods. Consume these no less than 30 minutes before meals and one hour after meals.

d) Eat organic whenever and as often as possible (refer to the Dirty Dozen at www.ewg.org). Otherwise try to buy locally grown fruits and vegetables in season. Wash all fruits and vegetables with mild dish soap and rinse thoroughly before eating.

e) Buy unsulphured dried fruit only. These can be found at health food stores. Ask for unsulphured if not clearly marked on package.

f) Always read the ingredients on every food package before you buy it. (*please refer to our Tips for Understanding Ingredient Labels in the following Diet section*)

g) Drink plenty of filtered water daily, approximately 6-8 glasses per day.

Coming off the diet: Reintroduce a new food with each meal and notice any reactions that result by keeping an accurate log of your results. This may include a reoccurrence of old symptoms, decreased energy levels and an obscured thinking process. You can test yourself through the slow introduction of foods. If you do notice changes in your health after reintroducing foods, you should be tested for food sensitivities and be treated with the Eliminate Allergy Technique (E.A.T.). If you notice no change in your health, you may not have food sensitivities and do not need to be tested for them.

Healthy Eating Habits: THE SEVEN STEP PLAN

1. Eliminate all "funky foods": All sugars, starches such as potatoes, white flour, white rice, caffeine and alcohol.

2. Eat fruit alone and on an empty stomach

3. Eat proteins (such as meat and eggs) and fats (such as butter and cheese) with vegetables.

4. Eat carbohydrates such as whole-grain pasta, with vegetables.

5. Do not eat proteins and fats with carbohydrates

6. Wait three hours between meals if switching from a protein/fat meal to a carbohydrate meal or vice versa.

7. Do not skip meals. Eat at least three a day and eat until you feel comfortably full.

Definitions

Organic: grown without the use of synthetic pesticides, herbicides, fungicides, petrochemically derived fertilizers, fumigants etc. and without being irradiated

Pasture-fed/Grass-fed: the animal has been raised outdoors and grass-fed. Some organic grain (like corn) may have been given as feed but the animal was pasture-fed during a large portion of its life. No antibiotics and/or carcinogenic hormones are given to the animal or included in its diet.

This diet has been composed expressly for the patients of NaturoMedic.com. All others who follow this diet do so at their own risk. Consult your primary health care provider about the applicability of such a diet in your particular case. (*please read the Diet for more information*)

Cholesterol

The soft, fat-like substance found in each cell of the body and in the bloodstream can be a sneaky culprit. Although your body makes all the cholesterol it requires, excess can accumulate from diet, increased weight, lack of physical activity, family history, smoking and certain medications. To reduce your cholesterol it is time to increase the "good" and lower the "bad". Understanding the differences between HDL and LDL will help you on your path to success.

LDL: Low Density Lipoprotein

- carry cholesterol from the liver to cells of the body
- excess LDL accumulate in artery walls forming a plaque and narrowing arteries when mixed with fat (atherosclerosis)

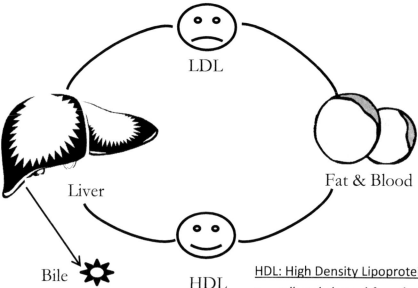

Bile:

- highest concentration of cholesterol in the body
- 94% recycled (bind up with diet recommendations to prevent recycling)

HDL: High Density Lipoprotein

- collect cholesterol from the body's tissues, and take it back to the liver
- scavenges and removes LDL
- transports LDL to liver to be reprocessed and passed from the body
- keeps inner walls of blood vessels clean

To Reduce Bad LDL (Low-Density Lipoprotein) Cholesterol

Oat bran is highly recommended for binding and removing excess cholesterol from the body. Additional LDL lowering foods include: oatmeal and dried beans, including plain baked beans out of the can. Soybeans (organic) are great for reducing genetically induced high cholesterol at any age. Grapefruit (segments and membrane, not the juice) drives down cholesterol. Fresh oranges, apples, yogurt, skim milk, carrots, garlic, onions, barley, ginger, eggplant, artichoke, unripe plantain, shiitake mushrooms and olive oil beneficially reduce cholesterol. Substitute seafood, including shellfish, for meat and chicken. Strawberries and bananas are high in the cholesterol reducing complex carbohydrate, pectin.

To Raise Good HDL (High-Density Lipoprotein) Cholesterol

Strong, raw onions are excellent HDL raising food. Try to have at least a half a medium onion per day. Substitute olive oil for other vegetable oils and saturated fats. Have alcoholic drinks, such as wine, beer and spirits in moderation (one or two drinks a day can boost HDL's). Remember to drink responsibly!

Additional Suggestions

Strictly limit total fat, especially saturated fats like animal-type fats, coconut and palm oils as they counteract the effects of the above natural cholesterol-fighters.

Cholesterol Rich Foods

1. For a low cholesterol diet restrict cholesterol to 50-100 g per day.
2. For a moderately low cholesterol diet restrict cholesterol to 100-150 g per day.

The following lists contain increased levels of cholesterol.

Very high amounts of cholesterol: 150-2000mg/100g edible portion:

- Brains
- Butter
- Caviar
- Egg yolk
- Whole egg
- Heart
- Kidney
- Liver
- Lobster
- Oysters
- Sweetbreads (thymus)

High amounts of cholesterol: 50-150mg/100g edible portion

- Beef
- Cheddar cheese
- Cream cheese
- Hard cheeses
- Cheese spread
- Chicken
- Crab
- Fish
- Lamb
- Lard and other animal fat
- Margarine (animal fat and vegetable fat combined)
- Mutton
- Pork
- Shrimp
- Veal

Moderate amounts of cholesterol: up to 50mg/100g edible portion

- Cottage cheese
- Low-fat cheese
- Ice cream
- Milk

References:
1. http://www.heart.org/HEARTORG/Conditions/Cholesterol/AboutCholesterol/Good-vs-Bad-Cholesterol_UCM_305561_Article.jsp
2. http://watchlearnlive.heart.org/CVML_Player.php?moduleSelect=hdlldl

Diet

Allergenic Foods and Food Sensitivities

Even though a food is classified as "healthy" or being a good source of nutrition, it does not mean that everyone can freely consume it without consequences. People can have an allergy or intolerance to many nutrient rich foods.

At NaturoMedic.com every patient is given a diet diary on his/her first visit to help the ND understand what you are eating. Many are not aware of what they consume and how food can have a dramatic effect on one's health. The diet diary includes a symptom column to bring patterns and associations with foods to light. Common ailments such as asthma, allergies, eczema, headaches, fatigue, bloating, gas and gastro-intestinal upset of any kind are directly affected by certain foods. It can be difficult to tell which foods are a problem because your body may be constantly overwhelmed with a chronic low-grade reaction-this has become your "normal". In order to determine the common offenders elimination diets are the next step. Foods that can trigger many health problems, (for example "the five white sins": white flour (breads and pastas), sugar, salt, fat (bad fats) and dairy are removed from the diet. Citrus (lemon is usually ok), wheat products, food additives and colorings can also create problems.

The Cleansing Diet used at NaturoMedic.com temporarily eliminates the most common problem foods from the diet for 5-10 days, giving the body an opportunity to rest. Many will notice a significant change in how they feel and a relief of symptoms. Foods are reintroduced one at a time. One food item per day is consumed at each meal. During the reintroduction period, if you have a re-occurrence of symptoms or the appearance of new symptoms, you most likely have a food sensitivity to that item. Think of your body with all its symptoms as being like a dirty kitchen floor; if you add more dirt, the kitchen floor it is still dirty. On the other hand, if you add dirt to a spotless kitchen floor, you will immediately see the dirt. The cleansing diet "cleans" out the body so we can see what is really happening. If certain foods are causing symptoms, the patient should be tested and treated for food sensitivities using the Eliminate Allergy Technique (EAT).

Gluten Free Diet

Gluten Foods	Gluten Free Alternatives
Wheat	Quinoa
Spelt	Buckwheat
Kamut	Millet
Barley	Amaranth
Rye	Chickpea flour
Oats (usually contaminated with other grains)	Almond meal
	Coconut flour
Found in: baking powder, pasta, cottage cheese, soy sauce, marshmallows, stamp adhesive, malt, many emulsifiers and flavorings.	Flax
	Potato flour
	Rice

Gluten is a protein found in many grains, especially wheat. Celiac disease is a condition where gluten cannot be tolerated in the diet. The gluten causes an autoimmune reaction in the intestines making it difficult to absorb nutrients. As many as 1 in 133 people are diagnosed with Celiac disease in Canada. It is also possible to be sensitive to gluten and not have Celiac disease; this is referred to as often gluten intolerance. Common symptoms associated with gluten intolerance or Celiac are: gas, bloating, pain, diarrhea, nausea, acid reflux, fatigue, anemia, tingling and numbness in the legs, etc.

Dairy Free Diet

Milk Ingredients to Watch For	Dairy Alternatives
Casein	Rice milk
Lactalbumin	Almond milk
Lactoglobulin	Hemp milk
Bovine albumin	Coconut milk
Gamma globulin	Soy milk (also a common allergen)
Milk solids	
Skim milk powder	
Caseinates	
Whey	
Albumin	

After infancy we are generally not well suited to consume milk. More than 7 million Canadians (20%) lack the enzymes to break down milk sugar, a condition known as lactose intolerance. In South Eastern Asia, lactose intolerance is

205

prevalent in 100% of Asians. Native Americans are 90% intolerant, South Americans, other Asians and most Africans are 50% lactose intolerant. The lowest prevalence is in North Western Europe and Scandinavia where the populations are 3-8% lactose intolerant. In the Mediterranean the prevalence rises to 70%. Milk contains many allergenic proteins such as casein. Common complaints associated with dairy intolerance include gas, bloating, diarrhea, constipation, gastro-intestinal bleeding, anemia, nausea and vomiting, acid reflux, headaches/migraines, joint pain or arthritis, ear infections, hay fever, asthma, eczema, ADHD and bedwetting in children.

Convenience Foods Allowed on the Cleansing diet	
Brown rice cracker, brown rice cakes	Apple butter, almond butter
Veggies cut up	Rice noodle dishes (Thai for example)
Hummus	Rice pasta dishes

When You Cannot Buy Organic

For vegetables: Avoid the 'dirty dozen' and consume foods with the least contamination *(please refer to the Pesticides for more information)*. Remember to thoroughly wash your foods with soap or with a vegetable wash from your local supermarket or health food store.

For Meat: Buy lean cuts of pesticide free meats. Trim the fat as the majority of the chemicals from pesticides are stored in the fatty parts of the animal.

If You Are Pressed For Time

Make recipes in large batches on your days off and freeze extra portions for readymade meals. Soups, stews, chili and brown rice can be cooked in larger quantities and used for a few days after. A slow cooker is another great way to save time and make food in advance.

Steaming Veggies

A gentle way to cook vegetables and retain most of the nutrients is steaming. Add an expandable steamer insert to any pot or purchase a steamer pot with a perforated insert. Lightly steam the vegetables to a crisp-tender consistency to maintain maximum nutrients. Reuse the water in soups for added vitamins. You can buy parchment paper in rolls like aluminum foil or in ready-made bags to wrap up veggies, fish, herbs and spices for readymade meals. Place the fresh raw ingredient in the bag or wrap it in the paper so the steam cannot escape and put in the oven. It is a quick method to cook and an easy clean-up too.

Tips for understanding ingredients labels

The following information was referenced from www.naturalnews.com:

1. Remember that ingredients are listed in order of their proportion in the product. This means the first 3 ingredients matter far more than anything else. The top 3 ingredients are what you are primarily eating.

2. If the list of ingredients contains long, chemical-sounding words that you cannot pronounce, avoid that item. It likely contains various toxic chemicals. Make sure you can recognize each ingredient.

3. When it comes to flour, wheat can be misleading. All flour derived from wheat can be called "wheat flour," even if it is processed, bleached and stripped of its nutrition. Only "whole grain wheat flour" is a healthful form of wheat flour. (Many consumers mistakenly believe that "wheat flour" products are whole grain products. In fact, this is not the case).

4. Be aware of serving sizes. For example, 2 chips have blank calories, but who really eats two chips? Food manufacturers can and do use this tactic to seemingly reduce the number of calories, grams of sugar or grams of fat in the package.

5. Certain **brown** products are not healthier than **white** products. Brown sugar is just white sugar with brown coloring and flavoring added, unless it is 100% natural brown sugar. Brown bread may not be healthier than white bread, unless it is made with whole grains.

6. Be conscious of where products that use herbs as an added health benefit are on the ingredient list. Some foods that include "goji berries" towards the end of the list actually contain very small amounts. A good product that really wants to use this herb will be listed closer to the front.

7. Remember that **ingredients lists do not have to list chemical contaminants**. Foods can be contaminated with pesticides, solvents, acrylamides, PFOA, perchlorate (rocket fuel) and other toxic chemicals without needing to list them at all. The best way to minimize your ingestion of toxic chemicals is to buy organic, or go with fresh, minimally-processed foods.

8. Look for words like "sprouted" or "raw" to indicate a higher-quality of natural foods. Sprouted grains and seeds are far healthier than non-sprouted. Raw ingredients are generally healthier than processed or cooked. Whole grains are healthier than "enriched" grains.

LABEL CLAIM	DEFINITION (per standard serving size)
Fat-free* or sugar-free	Less than 0.5 gram (g.) of fat or sugar
Low fat	3 g. of fat or less
Reduced fat or reduced sugar	At least 25% less fat or sugar
Cholesterol free	Less than 2 milligrams (mg.) cholesterol and 2 g. or less of saturated fat
Reduced cholesterol	At least 25% less cholesterol and 2 g. or less of saturated fat
Calorie free	Less than 5 calories
Low calorie	40 calories or less
Light or lite	1/3 fewer calories or 50% less fat

For more tips and recipes refer to the **NaturoMedic.com Healthy Living Cookbook**. You can download a free pdf copy from the following link http://naturomedic.com/

Kitchen Tools for Healthy Living

Minimum Equipment	Equipment to Make Life Easy
10 inch chef's knife	Food processor
Paring knife	Rice cooker
10 inch frying pan	Slow cooker
3 quart sauce pan	Baking pans (glass or stoneware)
Expandable steamer insert	Whisks
8-10 quart stock pot with a lid	Long handled Forks and tongs
Electric blender, or immersion blender	Mixing bowls
Roasting pan	Salad spinner
Liquid and dry measuring cups	Citrus juicer
Strainer	Garlic press
Hand grater, wooden spoons, rubber spatulas, vegetable peeler	Coffee grinder
	Serrated knife
* You want your pots and pans to be stainless steel, or ceramic lined instead of Teflon or aluminum, look for deals at discount or professional outlets, or restaurant supply stores.	Jars or glass containers for storage
	Cast iron skillet
	Juicer

Remember the 21-day rule to make a new habit and the 20-second rule to ensure your chance of ongoing successful changes (*please refer to Changing Habits*).

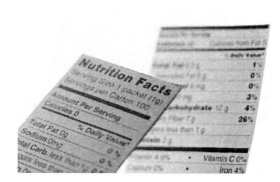

References:

1. www.celiac.com
2. www.gluten.org
3. http://www.foodreactions.org/intolerance/lactose/prevalence.html
4. http://www.hc-sc.gc.ca/fn-an/food-guide-aliment/using-utiliser/label-etiquet-eng.php
5. http://www.naturalnews.com/024414_food_fat_foods.html
6. http://www.mayoclinic.com/health/nutrition-facts/NU00293
7. http://www.naturalnews.com/
8. http://women.webmd.com/how-to-read-food-label

Therapeutic Fasting

Fasting is one of the oldest known health therapies. Throughout history, various cultures and religions have embraced the value of therapeutic fasting. Ancient Greek literature, the Koran and the Bible all make various references to fasting. The Bible mentions fasting on 74 different occasions. Moses fasted forty days and nights before receiving the Ten Commandments and Jesus fasted 40 days in the desert prior to starting his ministry. Hippocrates, the father of medicine, routinely recommended prolonged fasting. Pythagoras (c582-c500), a famous Greek philosopher, would not accept a potential student until they had fasted for 40 days. Even Benjamin Franklin often proposed that "the best of all medicines are rest and fasting." Evidently the benefits of a fast have been recognized for thousands of years.

Although research exists from the late 1800s on fasting, it remains a subject of limited study within the medical and scientific community. Fasting typically refers to the abstinence from food and drink except water for a specific period of time. But there are many variations depending upon the goal of the fast. There are fruit fasts, juice fasts and vegetable fasts. The fasting process spares the essential tissues (e.g. vital organs) while utilizing non-essential tissue (e.g. fat) for fuel. Alternatively, starvation utilizes essential tissue for energy. During starvation, the body uses protein from organs and muscles to function, since fat stores have been depleted. The following figure describes the stages of fasting.

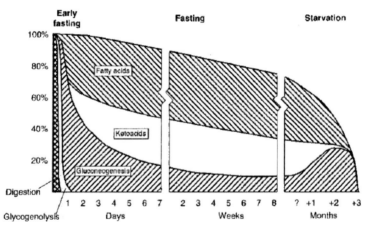

Figure 50-1 Energy reserve utilization during fasting.

Pizzorno, J. & Murray M. Textbook of Natural Medicine. 3rd edition. 2006. Elsevier Ltd. Churchill, Livingstone. p.g. 537

Stage 1: Early Fasting

Glucose (sugar) is synthesized by the liver during the initial lack of food. The liver stores of glycogen are depleted in the first few hours to make glucose (glycogenolysis). Afterwards glucose is generated (gluconeogenesis) from amino acids in the liver and muscle.

Stage 2: Fasting

Fatty acids (triglycerides) are the main energy source during fasting. Certain metabolic processes however do require amino acids for fuel causing protein stores to be broken down. A 160-pound man could safely fast for up to 2-3 months before starvation sets in.

Stage 3: Starvation

Once fat reserves are depleted and significant protein is used for energy production starvation can result. Protein stores are adequate for only a few weeks (gluconeogenesis). Eventually essential proteins are utilized and death can occur. Food is required after maximum fasting period (several weeks to months, dependent upon fat stores, metabolism and activity) to prevent Stage 3.

Research has shown the benefit of therapeutic fasting for a variety of conditions including: diabetes, high blood pressure, obesity, cardiovascular disease, dermatological ailments, gastrointestinal disorders, arthritis, allergies, mental illness and chemical poisoning.

- At the University of Minnesota in 1950, 32 volunteers fasted for 8 months. In comparison to food deprivation cases during World War II, the observations confirmed that the fasting period did not lead to any deficiencies in vitamins or minerals. Improvements did occur in diabetes and skin ailments.

- Fasting alone was recommended in the treatment of mild to moderate acute pancreatitis following a random trial of 88 patients in 1984.

- In 1984, the American Journal of Industrial Medicine studied patients who had ingested rice oil contaminated with PCB's (polychlorinated biphenyls). Following a 7-10 day fast, subjects reported symptom improvement. Caution was noted with patients known to suffer from significant contamination of fat-soluble toxins as toxic levels may be reached in the bloodstream. (i.e. DDT, dichlorodiphenyltrichloroethane, is mobilized into blood during a fast and may lead to toxic levels to the nervous system).

- In 1991, Dr. Jan Palmblad MD, PhD. concluded in the Nutrition and Rheumatoid Disease journal that "total fasting may be the most rapid and available means of inducing relief of arthritic pain and swelling for those who have rheumatoid arthritis. It can be done with a minimum of

211

discomfort and safely if not prolonged more than one week. The mechanisms of the beneficial effects of fasting still remain to be discovered. Immune anti-inflammatory systems are changed by fasting."

- Further literature has suggested the benefit of fasting to: eczema, psoriasis, IBS, depression, schizophrenia, ulcers, fibroids, autoimmune disease, etc.

What can be expected during a fast?

Fasts are individualized and can vary in length from 3 to 7 days. In general, in the first 1-15 days as the body uses up glucose, hypoglycemic reactions can occur. The severity can vary and symptoms may range from nothing at all to feeling lightheaded or faint to mood swings, to headaches and body aches.

After glucose stores have been exhausted and the body begins to mobilize fat, the extent of fat soluble toxins present in the body will directly correspond to the symptoms experienced. The majority of harmful materials are either fat or water-soluble. Water-soluble toxins are eliminated by the kidneys. The fat-soluble toxins are predominantly removed by the liver. The body is continuously exposed to chemicals in food as preservatives and stabilizers or as pesticides on the surface of fruits and vegetables. Pesticides and herbicides are generally fat soluble so they attach to the plant and do not wash off in the rain (water-soluble). The fat-soluble toxins concentrated in the liver and cells are mobilized during the fast. The greater the amounts the more prolonged and severe your symptoms may be. Feeling ill from detoxification could last for 2 to 5 days depending upon the fast. The symptoms during toxin elimination are equivalent to a healing crisis.

Imagine your blood with food molecules in it. As you start fasting the food molecules are consumed. The cells without food utilize the stored glucose and then metabolize fat for fuel, simultaneously mobilizing fat soluble toxins. Initially the liver and kidneys are overwhelmed by the burden placed on them (the bodies symptoms of brain fog, headaches, bloating and pain are all a reflection of this). Once the liver and kidneys begin to catch up, symptoms subside, energy increases, mental clarity improves and there is frequently a strong sense of well-being. A feeling of euphoria is often expressed from those who chose to meditate or pray during their healing journey (this is commonly the religious benefit of fasting). Supplements are prescribed to accelerate the detox process in order to achieve faster results.

There is often a concern of whether sensations of hunger will be experienced throughout the fast. Intense hunger usually lasts for the first few days followed by almost no hunger at all. Incidentally, those who attach a high social and psychological stigma to food can find the fast quite difficult.

Therapeutic fasting is advantageous for disease management and prevention. To attain optimal health fasting once a year for more than three days is recommended until good clarity of thought, energy stability and decreased symptoms are achieved. It is advised to consult a licensed practitioner well versed in fasting protocols for your first endeavor.

*must be a patient of NaturoMedic.com in order to receive treatment protocol

References:
1. Pizzorno, J. & Murray M. Textbook of Natural Medicine. 3rd edition. 2006. Elsevier Ltd. Churchill, Livingstone. pg. 533-545.
2. http://www.chuckrowtaichi.com/Fasting.html
3. Prytula, M. Therapeutic Fasting. NaturoMedic.com. www.NaturoMedic.com. posted online Oct 2004.

NaturoMedic.com Weight Loss Tips

Losing weight is not a simple task. Taking a miracle pill and immediately losing all our excess weight would of course be ideal, but we all know that it does not work like that. Your body had to work to put on the weight and therefore you must work to take off the extra pounds. There are few tips and tricks you can use in order to help make weight loss easier for you.

The Mind

There is a neurological component strongly associated with weight gain. First, there is eating for emotional comfort. Appetite is the body's natural way to balance food consumption with energy expenditure to maintain a stable and healthy body weight. A number of different hormones signal the brain when food is needed or not. These signals are received by dopamine-producing neurons in the hypothalamus of the brain, modifying the brain's reward center and motivation for food. During periods of stress, sadness or grief, it is very common to eat in order to feel better. In some cases, emotional binging occurs. When we binge, we eat much larger quantities than we normally would and more than our bodies can handle. Unfortunately, this easily contributes to putting on the pounds. We eat more because the hormones responsible for controlling appetite become deregulated, specifically leptin and insulin. Leptin is released from fat cells to decrease appetite when the body has had enough. Insulin suppresses appetite when blood sugar is high. When these hormones become unbalanced, dopamine levels in the reward center of the brain are elevated, triggering unnecessary and inappropriate hunger. Binge eating also leads more food cravings and less satisfaction, similar to the diminishing pleasure alcoholics or drug addicts experience. Binge eating actually triggers the same dopamine response in the reward center as nicotine and cocaine. The 20-second rule can be employed to help with removal of processed food stuffs.

Second, weight gain is also a form of protection. We have all heard of building a wall around us; we keep our feelings inside and become closed off from others. We can also build this wall physically. Our mind feels the need to keep us safe from the stresses we are facing in our lives and so the switch to turn off our hunger is overridden and we continue to eat to feel secure. With extra weight, people cannot get as close to you. Our mind is very strong. While it can help protect us emotionally and physically, it can also play tricks on us. It is not easy for the body to let go of the extra weight. We go to the gym and eat less, but nothing happens. In our mind, we are still threatened by the stresses in our lives and letting go of the weight will make us vulnerable, so the mind will hold onto the weight. Once we begin to deal with these conflicts and build security, the weight will start to come off. Some women feel threatened by undue sexual energy directed towards them and they may put on weight just to stop it. Men may have felt bullied when they were younger, so the excess weight gain makes it harder to be pushed around.

Hunger and Thirst

The connection the mind has to the body is very real. As discussed above, emotional eating can easily turn off the signal that we are full. The mind can suppress our 'stop eating' mechanism. After a while we begin to eat because we think we should and not necessarily because we are hungry. Your body needs to relearn what hunger is. Next time you think about eating, take a moment and make sure that you are truly hungry. You do not have to skip any meals, but you may notice that you do not have to snack as often. Knowledge is power. Learn to recognize true hunger vs. emotional eating). As we said the mind can be tricky. The mind can also confuse thirst with hunger. Often times we feel hungry so we go for a snack, but in fact what the body really wants is fluid. Relearning the difference between thirst and hunger is something we may also need to do. When you do feel hungry, before reaching for a snack, try having a glass of water first to see if that corrects the problem. Eventually your mind and body will be able to distinguish between the two.

Am I Full?

As you can tell, resetting the body and mind connection is very important with weight loss. The next step is taking the time to enjoy your food. Living in a high paced society, we have grown accustomed to eating on the go and eating quickly. Did you know that it takes 20 minutes for your stomach to tell your brain that it is full? Eating quickly can lead to second helpings and overfilling the stomach before the mind can tell you to stop. Ever feel too full once you are done eating? This is because, by the time you stop eating, the stomach has already expanded beyond its optimal capacity and now needs to work harder. Taking 20 minutes to enjoy a meal can let the brain know you have had enough and allow it to turn off the hunger signal. Learning to take your time to eat may take a few days. Some tips that may help are:

1. Chew slowly. Try not to eat quickly, chew each bite. Counting a certain number of chews per bite helps prepare your food for proper digestion for the stomach (e.g. minimum 15 chews per bite).

2. Pause in between bites and put your fork down while you are chewing.

3. Try eating with your opposite hand. It will not only take longer, but you will definitely have a good laugh. You may even become ambidextrous. If necessary sit on your eating hand.

Positive Food Environment

Like emotions, our environment can play a role in our eating habits. Eating while watching television or a movie can actually cause you to eat more. We eat faster as we get more involved with the program and pay less attention to what and how much we are eating. Sit at the table away from the TV, computers or talking on the phone. Pay attention to your food and enjoy it. Put your taste buds to work. Surround yourself with positive conversation at the table and avoid any negative topics until after you are done eating.

Make a Plate

What we put on our plate is very important to eating a proper diet, maintaining blood sugar and balancing our appetite. Protein is essential for the body to keep insulin levels normalized and prevent them from spiking. Elevated levels of insulin over time lead to weight gain and insulin resistance (contributing to type II diabetes). Fiber will help to curb your appetite, keep you full for longer periods and is essential for the proper functioning of the digestive system. Preparing your plate for each meal is a necessary step.

1. Select a small dinner plate. Contemporary plate styles are quite large and look great but are very misleading about portion sizes. Filling a smaller plate looks better and is more appealing to our tricky brain.

2. Fill your plate with the appropriate portions of protein, carbohydrate and vegetables. Your plate should resemble the following diagram.

Protein (25%)

Carbohydrate (25%)

Vegetables (50%)

3. Remember to wait 20 minutes before going for seconds. If you are still hungry, then have more vegetables or a little bit of everything. Do not refill the plate with the same amount.

Portion Sizes

Every person has a different body type and does not require the same amount of food or nutrients. Your body can actually tell you how much you should be eating. Use your hand as a guide when you set up a plate to determine your individual portion sizes.

1. Protein: equivalent to the palm of your hand

2. Carbohydrates: make a fist.

    - Loose fist for complex carbohydrate

    - Tight fist for simple carbohydrate

3. Veggies: open up your hand nice and wide. This is one portion not to skimp on.

Make a habit

Remember it takes 21 days to introduce a new habit. Be patient and stick with it! (see Changing Habits section).

Weight loss is a multifactorial approach and many factors need to be addressed. Important factors that can also be addressed are:

Blood sugar
Exercise
Pop
Alcohol
Stress
MRT

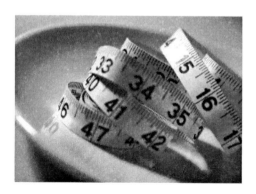

Chapter 10

NaturoMedic.com Treatments

*must be a patient of NaturoMedic.com in order to receive treatment protocol

Botanical Medicine

The earliest written records of nearly all civilizations mention the use of herbs for healing. Emperor Shen Nung (3494 B.C) tasted various plants to determine their medicinal properties. Poisoning himself 100 times, his trial and error method contributed to the discovery of medicinal plants throughout the world. The World Health Organization estimates that 80% of the world's population presently uses herbal medicine for some aspect of primary health care. The United States 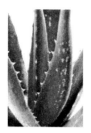 National Cancer Institute has identified 3,000 plants from which anticancer drugs are made from. Modern medicine draws its origins from early herbal therapies. Until the past 100 years, all MDs prescribed herbs routinely.

The development of synthetic medicine signalled the decline of MDs using herbs directly. Chemists began to isolate active ingredients in plants and to learn how to produce the component independently of the herb. In 2001, researchers identified 122 compounds used in mainstream medicine which were derived from plant sources. At least 7,000 medical compounds in the modern pharmacopoeia that are derived from plants. For example, Salicin, the analgesic component of aspirin, is derived from the bark of the White Willow *(Salix alba)*. Newly synthesised compounds would have a similar chemical structure as the natural ingredient but are more potent, more dangerous and more likely to lead to profound toxic effects. These effects were labelled as "side effects", but they are really the normal action of the synthetic active ingredient in the body merely acting in ways other than intended. For example, gastrointestinal disturbances are very common with aspirin. This side effect is less likely to occur with the plant as the dose and the concentration are not as strong. With this new age of synthetic medicine came the development of new miracle drugs. It also saw an increase in disease from medication, side effects and adverse reactions. Many of us may be familiar with "take Drug A for your _____ and take Drug B to help with nausea that you will get from Drug A". Does this method of treatment truly seem logical?

Botanical medicine or preparations derived from the plant are usually safer and slower acting than drug therapy, resulting in less toxic effects. When using the plant directly, you are utilizing the active ingredient and all the associated factors in the plant. This makes the action of the particular ingredient more effective in its natural state as it works in conjunction with the other components. In fact the benefit of an herb is usually due to the total interaction of all its constituents and not just the active ingredient. Consequently, there are few herb-related diseases.

The safety of medication is of course very important. Any medicine can be toxic when used improperly. It is a common misconception that botanical medications are completely safe and nontoxic; natural does not always mean safe! Drug interactions can occur not only between the drugs. They can also occur between drugs and herbs, herbs and herbs, herbs and nutrients, nutrients and nutrients, etc. Knowledge of botanical toxicology is essential before attempting to treat with herbs. In general, botanical medicine is safer and more therapeutic than the use of drugs when prescribed appropriately, at correct dosages and monitored properly.

The majority of negative reactions between botanical herbs and drugs are predominantly due to an interaction with a particular ingredient in the herb with the drug. In many cases, regulating authorities fail to realize that a significant amount of the herb must be consumed in order to cause a negative interaction with the drug.

At NaturoMedic.com, your ND is fully trained in botanical medicine. Western botanicals are prescribed on an individual basis, combined in such a manner as to keep your medications at a minimum. They are formulated to aid in stimulating or directing your body's own healing forces, in order to isolate a disease causing factor and to promote health from within.

References:

1. Trattler, Better Health Through Natural Healing. McGraw-Hill, 1985.
2. Fabricant DS, Farnsworth NR (March 2001). The value of plants used in traditional medicine for drug discovery. *Environ. Health Perspect.* 109 Suppl 1: 69–75.
3. The World Health Organization: Traditional medicine Fact sheet N°134, 2008. www.who.int
4. Interactive European Network for Industrial Crops and their Applications (2000-2005). http://ec.europa.eu/research/quality-of-life/ka5/en/00111.html
5. Cragg G.M. & Newman D.J. Plants as a source of anti-cancer agents.Ethnopharmacology vol. I
6. Tierra, M. The Way of Chinese Herbs. 1998. Pocket Books, New York, NY.

BioClimate Reprogramming

Exposure to the elements can wreak havoc on the body and cause a multitude of ailments. Evidence has demonstrated a direct connection between temperature and migraines, arthritic pain and weather. From a Chinese Medicine perspective, the invasion of external disease causing factors can alter physiological processes and lead to complications. More specifically cold, heat, wind, dampness, dryness and darkness have all been identified as external elements to which one's body can become over sensitive and have a negative reaction to. Some examples of invasion and the body's possible responses are:

1. **Cold** invasion from walking through the frozen food isle.
    - Avoiding the isle for fear of feeling cold, catching a cold, shivering or experiencing hypothermia symptoms.
2. **Cold** invasion from drinking a cold drink on a hot day.
    - Easily experiencing prolonged brain shock or brain freeze.
3. **Wind** invasion from driving with the windows down.
    - Being aggravated with aches, pains or stiffness in the ears, neck or shoulders. Commonly suffering from colds.
4. **Heat** invasion from being outside on a warm, humid day.
    - Remaining cool and indoors to avoid feeling faint, lightheaded, swollen or sinus congested.
5. **Dark** invasion from the winter months where days are shorter and sunless.
    - Feeling sad, depressed and moody – overall, feeling mentally unwell. (Seasonal Affective Disorder)

Throughout these examples there is an apparent emotional component attached to the disease factor. The subconscious is a powerful ally, designed to protect you. Negative subconscious processes that interfere with life and potentiate symptoms can also be masked by the mind's survival safeguard. The goal of BioClimate Reprogramming (BCR) is to erase negative subconscious programs attached to the various external factors.

Qi is known as your vital force in Traditional Chinese Medicine. It is equivalent to the *Vis* from Chapter 2. It is important for your vital force to flow freely throughout the body without impediment. It plays a role in defending the body from pathogens, regulating growth and development, ensuring blood circulation and maintaining overall homeostasis. Invasion from an external disease factor can constrict and trap your energy. Contributing to any imbalances and enhancing symptoms. These can range from fatigue, dizziness, shortness of breath, abdominal discomfort, digestive disorders, joint pain, muscle spasms, arthritis to various skin conditions. In addition to removing subconscious patterns associated with disease, BCR can remove blockages and help *Qi* move smoothly throughout the body.

BCR treatments do more than simply desensitize you to the climate; they work to remove the invasion.

Potential Symptoms of Cold Invasion
- Overall cold feeling
- Body chills
- Body aches
- Muscle Cramps
- Feeling worse in cold weather
- Disliking air conditioning
- 'Brain freeze' that occurs easily (e.g. from cold drinks or food)
- Needing a sweater for warmth (i.e. when walking through frozen food isle)
- Raynaud's or decreased circulation
- Asthma
- Abdominal Conditions–Irritable bowel syndrome, bloating, constipation etc.
- Arthritis (mixture of cold and damp invasion)
- Failing muscular coordination
- Slurred speech
- Blurred vision
- Shuffling small steps
- Irrational behavior

Interestingly, symptoms are very similar to hypothermia, dementia and Parkinson's disease

Potential Symptoms of Heat Invasion
- Sensitive to humid days (combination of hot damp invasion)
  o Headaches
  o Sinus Congestion
  o Dizziness/Light Headedness
  o Fainting
- Menopause
- Excessive Sweating
- Skin Conditions (e.g. eczema, acne rosacea)
- Multiple Sclerosis (disease factor can vary per person)

Potential Symptoms of Wind Invasion

- Rheumatism pains that move around and are never the same
- Headaches
- Earaches
- Facial nerve damage (Bell's Palsy)
- Sensitive to drafts (e.g. work or sleep in an area where a breeze is constantly blowing on you)

Potential Symptoms of Dark Invasion

- Depression/sadness
- Anxiety/fear
- Insomnia/sleep disorders
- PTSD – post traumatic stress disorder.
- Panic attacks
- Heart attacks

The section about our subconscious, demonstrated the brain's natural tendency to ensure survival. Upon exposure to an external disease factor the subconscious automatically searches for previous programs to tell it how to react. For example, in Raynaud's Disease, the body will shunt blood away from the hands to the core upon exposure to the cold. These old programs may have served us well once but the subconscious does not know if this is a good or bad program. It simply knows it ensured your survival. Cold is the most potentially life threatening of the external disease factors. The nervous system is hardwired to respond to cold immediately as it can be lethal quickly. With less than 1 minute exposure to cold, our bodies react, by trying to warm up the cold area. Exposure over 1 minute results in the body responding by going into hypothermia protection mode. Heat is the second most life-threating of the external disease causing factor. Heat exposure of up to 5 minutes is very stimulating to circulation while greater than 5 minutes our bodies go into hyperthermia protection mode.

NaturoMedic.com will seek to assess which external factor has invaded and determine the appropriate BioClimate Reprogramming therapy. BCR has the capacity to remove disease, decrease symptoms, erase negative programs, eliminate *Qi* blockages and desensitize your nervous system to the elements.

Chelation

What is Chelation?

Chelation is most commonly referred to as the activity of a synthetic amino acid encapsulating heavy metals and minerals and making it possible for the body to excrete them. Chele is latin for claw. A chelator (EDTA, DMSA, DMPS, and others) binds to a heavy metal in a pincer like grasp, pulling them out of the tissues and into the blood for removal through the urine.

Is Chelation a New Therapy for Heart Disease and Hypertension?

Physicians administering chelation for lead toxicity observed that patients who also had atherosclerosis (fatty-plaque buildup on arterial walls) or arteriosclerosis (hardening of the arteries) experienced reductions in both conditions after chelation. Since 1952, IV EDTA chelation has been used to treat cardiovascular disease.

How does it Work?

Chelation therapy involves the injection or oral administration of chelating agents into the bloodstream for the purpose of eliminating undesirable substances from the body. These include heavy metals, chemical toxins, mineral deposits, and fatty plaques (as in the arteries; the agent binds to the calcium in the plaques). EDTA, DMPS and DMSA are widely studied effective chelating agents.

What is the purpose of EDTA?

- Chelation is similar to ice dissolving in a glass of water (slowly one molecule at a time so you cannot even see it happen) rather than being broken off like a jack hammer breaking up concrete. (John Parks Towbridge, MD, FACAM, Manual of the Intl. Society of Chelation Technicians)
- Toxic metals are the greatest source of oxidative damage in the body. Antioxidants are used to combat this damage. If the biggest source of oxidative damage in the body is removed then less antioxidants are needed.
- Chelates or removes toxic metals, including aluminum and **lead**.
- Removes lead which destroys endothelial cells (cells on the inner most lining of blood vessels). These cells release nitric oxide which dilates the blood vessel to increase blood flow.
- Lowers serum ionized calcium, which decreases clotting and reduces spasm.
- Reduces LDL cholesterol content in the liver and arterial plaque.
- Chelation therapy is given in a physician's office as an intravenous infusion over 30 minutes-3 hours, depending on the chelator.
- Can be given by injection

What is the purpose of DMPS?

- Very specific chelator of mercury (body)

What is the purpose of DMSA?

- Given orally
- Chelates arsenic, cadmium, lead, mercury (brain), nickel, tin and uranium
- Safe for adults and children
- Stephanie Cave, M.D.–reported safety and efficacy from over 2700 patients: "DMSA treatment has been a pivotal point in the treatment for many children in the autism spectrum"

Benefits of Chelation and Resulted Improvement in Function of:

- Kidneys
- Immune System
- Lungs -90.5% improvement in pulmonary function
- Vision
- Energy
- Digestion
- Improved circulation all over the body. Intra-arterial obstruction decreased by 20.9% (± 2.3%)

Reduced Risk of:

- Stroke
- Heart Attack
- Cancer-after 18 years, 1.7% of EDTA treated patients died of cancer while 17.6% of untreated patients died of cancer
- Arthritis

No deaths have been reported in the medical literature attributed to chelation therapy using the ACAM (American College for Advancement in Medicine) protocol.

Cost Effectiveness:

- According to Hancke's data EDTA treatments might have prevented 363,000 of the 407,000 bypass procedures done in the US in 1991, saving more than $8 billion dollars.
- Arteries become softer and more flexible, allowing increased blood flow throughout the body.
- Increasing the diameter of an artery by 15% will double the blood flow through the artery.
- The goal of therapy is to restore normal function.

Interesting Statistics:

- 58 out of 65 patients on the waiting list for bypass surgery were able to cancel it after chelation therapy
- 2,870 patients were studied, using objective non-invasive measurements. There was marked and good improvement in:
  - Heart Patients-93.5%
  - Arteriosclerotic Vascular Disease of the Leg-98.5%
  - Brain Disorders-54.0%

Carotid Artery:

- EDTA chelation therapy was used to treat 30 patients with carotid artery blockage as measured objectively by Doppler imaging before and after 30 EDTA infusions over a 10-month period.
- Overall 30% reduction in plaque
- Severe stenosis had even greater reduction
- Clear evidence of reversal of atherosclerosis-improvements in 80-90% of patients with only 10 requiring surgical intervention

Vascular Disease:

EDTA chelation therapy related to improvement in vascular disease by objective testing before and after treatment.

- 19 articles met the criteria
- 22,765 patients
- 87% improved
- Correlation coefficient 0.88% (high)

EDTA and chelation work by removing heavy metals, *please refer to Heavy Metals for more information.*

Please Note: Abbott Labs Patent for EDTA expired in 1969. Manufacturers were directed to remove claims of chelation benefit in cardiovascular disease.

References:

1. Rudolph, C., McDonagh, E. & Barber, R. 1989. Effect of EDTA chelation and supportive multivitamin/trace mineral supplementation on chronic lung disorders: a study of FVC and FEV1. Journal of Advancement in Medicine. 2(4):553-561.
2. Blumer, W. & Cranton, W. 1989. Report on EDTA and Cancer.
3. Rudolph, C.J., McDonagh, E.W. & Barber, R.K. A nonsurgical approach to obstructive carotid stenosis using EDTA chelation. Journal of Advancement in Medicine. 1991;4(3):157-168.
4. Chappell, L. & Stahl, J. The correlation between EDTA chelation therapy and improvement in cardiovascular function: a meta-analysis. Journal of Advancement in Medicine. 1993;6(3):139-160.
5. Hancke, C. & Flytie K. Benefits of EDTA chelation therapy in arteriosclerosis: a retrospective study of 470 patients. Journal of Advancement in Medicine. 1993;6(3):161-171.

Chinese Herbal Patents

Chinese medicines are made from a variety of ingredients including roots, bark, leaves and flowers. These patented formulations may be used to treat many health conditions as they are constructed to correct specific imbalances in the body. Traditional Chinese Medicine has been used for over 5,000 years.

In the West, medicine is an analytical science, dissecting things until causal links are made. In Chinese medicine, the opposite occurs. Signs and symptoms are pieced together until a picture of the whole person appears. Treatment therefore is centered on the person rather than on the disease. In traditional Chinese medicine many factors and properties are considered in the diagnoses. For instance, an individual's vital force (also known as *Qi*) may be weak, leading to a susceptibility to attack from external pathogens. The flow of blood, the functioning of specific organs, temperature, taste and weather all play a role. These properties can also be treated, stimulated or tonifyed by particular herbs and substances. This concept of using herbs to correct particular functions in the body has been developed over generations.

In Chinese medicine, there are 5 external disease factors that can invade the body and effect organ function: wind, cold, heat, dryness and dampness. The therapeutic capabilities of a substance can be described by linking its taste and temperatures to disease causing factors. For example, a warm substance can be used for an externally contracted cold or a cool substance for heat. By understanding the properties of a substance, we can treat the cause of the organ imbalance. In addition, 5 internal disease factors directly correspond to organ pathology. Anxiety (worry), fear (fright), grief, joy (or absence of joy) and anger (depression) can impact the function of an organ and lead to a clinical presentation. Stress experienced on a daily basis cause excessive activity of the liver to overact on the stomach/spleen contributing to loose stools. Knowing which herb will work toward rebalancing the organs and emotions is critical. In fact, the effect that the substance has on the organ will depend on many factors including taste. A sweet herb tonifies the Spleen, an organ that prefers sweet, but the same herb may drain an organ with an aversion to this quality like the Heart. Herbs also have a directional tendency to rise, fall, float or sink. This is indicative of the situations in which it can be used effectively. Substances that rise move upward and outward, promoting sweating and dispersing cold, while substances that fall move downward redirecting rebellious *Qi* (e.g. vomiting) or preventing abnormal loss of fluids. The many therapeutic uses and the versatility of the herbs and substances can be combined to enhance their qualities, restore the body and jump start the patient's own healing powers.

At NaturoMedic.com, many of the herbs we use are commercially prepared patents that are packaged in China. These products offer, convenient and affordable treatment alternatives and are largely free of any side effects.

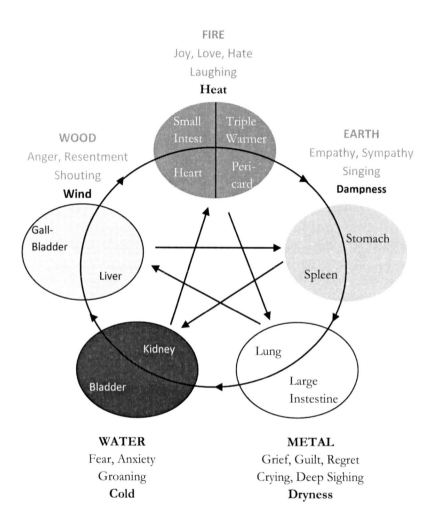

References:
1. Bensky & Gamble. Chinese Herbal Medicine. Chinese Herbal Medicine Materia Medica. Eastland Press.
2. Thie & Thie. Touch for Health; A Practical Guide to Natural Health with Acupressure Touch. Devorss Publications.

Colon Hydrotherapy

Colon therapy is a valuable procedure and treatment for a variety of colon conditions and as part of a fasting or cleansing program. A colonic treatment offers a gentle cleansing of the last five feet of the digestive tract. The purpose of the colon is to remove waste material from the body by mass muscular contractions called peristalsis. Colon therapy provides therapeutic improvement of muscular tone, which facilitates peristalsis and benefits the sluggish colon. Colonics also help reduce the transit time of waste, helping to stop the recycling of fat soluble toxins. Normally 94% of bile and fat soluble toxins are recycled. During a fast, on day's two to five, colon hydrotherapy is recommended to ensure the flushing of fat soluble toxins form the body. The effects of a stagnant colon can be manifested in the form of constipation, halitosis (bad breath), skin problems, headaches, low back pain, lack of energy and low sex drive. By stripping down biofilm (the old, toxic mucous lining of the bowel), a major source of disease in the body is removed. The bowel is then open to a more efficient means of eliminating waste and absorbing nutrients, both of which are essential to any lasting healing process.

The colon is approximately 5 to 5½ feet long. It contains the largest concentration of bacteria in the body. These beneficial bacteria help to synthesize important nutrients including folic acid, B vitamins and vitamin K. Waste material allowed to stagnate alters the proportion of healthy bacteria to disease producing bacteria, preventing proper elimination and absorption leading to toxic accumulation. When waste arrives at the inner walls of the colon from circulating blood, the buildup of feces prevents their removal. The colon becomes weak, waste materials accumulate and the colon becomes irritated. There are multiple causes that can affect proper bowel function: poor dietary habits, dehydration, illness, medications, emotional and physical stress. Restoring efficient bowel peristalsis and digestion is very important to your health.

Colonics: Before, During and After

1. **Preparing For Your Colonic**
- Drink plenty of water. If your system is not hydrated, the body tries to meet its need for water by absorption through the colon walls. This can slow the rate of release during the colonic.
- Do not eat anything 2 hours before a colonic (water and juice are ok).
- Avoid any gas forming foods the day before your colonic (i.e. beans, broccoli, cauliflower, cabbage, onions, cucumbers, pop).
- If fasting, continue on with your routine.

2. What to Expect During Your Colonic

- A colonic is a safe, gentle infusion of treated water into the colon via the rectum.

- The patient lies comfortably on a treatment table during the procedure with privacy being maintained during the entire session. A small disposable sterile speculum is gently inserted into the rectum through which warm water passes into the colon.

- The skilled therapist will use several "fills and releases" of water as well as gentle massage techniques to dislodge the toxic waste material adhering to the walls of the colon

- The waste is then gently washed away through the system's closed waste disposal hose. No mess, no odour.

Note: some people do not get a huge release. This could be due to elevated feelings of anticipation and nervousness surrounding the procedure. In addition people who already have 2-3 bowel movements per day may not have a large elimination. Pockets of gas can also block the flow of water into the colon during the procedure. Usually if you do not have any elimination during the procedure, you will have a successful elimination immediately afterwards. A small or no release of stool does not suggest that the treatment was unsuccessful as the colon is still being flushed of built up toxins.

3. Post Treatment

After your colonic, it is important to:

- Drink plenty of fluids (distilled water, juices, herb teas)
- Avoid eating raw vegetables for 2 days. Cooked or steamed vegetables are permitted

Replace Intestinal Flora:

- Acidophilus should be taken as indicated on the label

Avoid foods and beverages such as:

- Alcohol, caffeinated beverages, chocolate, dairy products, fatty and fried foods, sugar and wheat products.
- Gas producing vegetables such as beans, broccoli, Brussels sprouts, cabbage, onions, peppers and raw vegetables are also to be avoided
- Reduce meat consumption for 3 days (heavy pork and beef)
- If on a fast, continue on with the routine
- Observe your body closely for its reaction to the colonic, the food you eat and your energy level

- Be prepared that the colonic might precipitate a healing crisis. By releasing these toxins, energy in the body is available to help other areas

Most Important Organ in the Body:

"The Brain said I should be in charge, because without me nothing would happen. The Stomach said I should be in charge because I process all the food and give you all energy. The Eyes said I should be in charge because I allow the body to see. The Kidneys said I should be in charge because I clean and filter any toxins in the body. The Colon said I should be in charge, and before he could say why, all the other organs laughed and insulted him. "RIGHT"!! The colon was so upset that it decided to go on strike! Within a few days the brain had a terrible headache. The stomach was bloated. The kidneys were overworked. The blood had gone toxic. The eyes had double vision and gone blurry. They all agreed that the colon should be the boss."

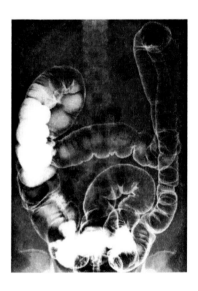

Colour Therapy

Colour therapy affects all levels of your being. When the body is not able to use light and function optimally, vitality and energy are lowered and the body is open to disease and decay.

Humans physically see light as a vibrational quality. The vibrational quality of colour can be used to reestablish the right frequency when there is too much or too little vibration in the body. Colour is very effective in healing due to its ability to reestablish and maintain balance in the body. When this balance is not evident, disease is allowed to begin. Colour therapy works to alleviate these blocks that cause disharmony in the body.

Contacts and glasses should not be worn during colour therapy treatment.

The 12 Colours and Their Relation to Your Well-Being

Blue: Sedates the nervous system. Acts to improve throat conditions, hoarseness, teething, fevers, measles, hysteria, palpitations, spasms, menstrual problems, acute rheumatism, shock, etc.

Green: Balances the brain, body and endocrine system. Acts to improve heart problems, blood pressure, ulcers, headaches and neuralgia.

Indigo: Nerve sedative and immune stimulant. Acts to support the parathyroid by toning down the thyroid and calms down respiration. A general sedative.

White: Balances and harmonizes the body and mind.

Orange: Stimulant. Acts to support and stimulate the lungs, stomach, spleen, pancreas and thyroid. Also acts as a decongestant and antispasmodic. Improves asthma, colds, bronchitis, rheumatism, epilepsy, gall stones, gout, menstrual problems, hyper or hypothyroidism, mental exhaustion and kidney ailments.

Red: Energizer. Acts to support the sensory nervous system. This system governs our five senses: sight, hearing, touch, taste and smell. Helps to counteract the effect of burns and also helps the liver and aids the body to increase platelets and hemoglobin.

Violet: Immune stimulant. Acts to support and stimulate the spleen. Promotes white blood cells. Calms muscular activity and overactive lymphatic glands.

Red/orange: Stimulates and energizes the organs and nervous system.

Yellow/green: Energizes while balancing the brain, body and endocrine system.

Ruby: General stimulant. Acts to stimulate the kidneys and adrenals. Strengthens arteries, raises blood pressure, raises heart rate and promotes rapid delivery at child birth.

Yellow: Energizer. Strengthens the nerves and aids the brain. Acts to support and stimulate the intestines, pancreas, digestive fluids and motor nerves, thereby helping to energize muscles. Yellow has a stimulating, cleaning and eliminating action on the liver, intestines and skin and is energizing to the alimentary tract. Useful in treating constipation, diabetes, flatulence, digestive problems, eczema, kidneys, mental depression, mental exhaustion, acute inflammation, over-excitement, liver problems, palpitation of the heart and paralysis.

Blue/green: Soother. Acts to calm down the brain, tone the skin and help balance your entire system.

Once the colour needed has been determined, then the desired strobe effect is chosen using muscle testing to reach the appropriate level of the mind. The four levels the body can use are:

- BETA: greater than 13Hz, used for the conscious level
- ALPHA: 8-12 Hz, used for learning and REM sleep
- THETA: 4-7- Hz, REM sleeping only
- DELTA: 1-3 Hz, Very deep sleep

Colour Therapy has many unique applications. It can be used as a standalone therapy or it can also be used in conjunction with other therapies such as MET, EAT and MRT, making them more effective.

What Personal Colour Preferences Tell About You
Psychological choices of colour tell a lot about a person and their state of health. For example:

- Outgoing people prefer warm colours
- Introverted or ego-centered people prefer cool colours, as they do not require other stimulation
- Emotionally responsive individuals react freely with colours
- Emotionally inhibited individuals often react strongly to colour, as it intrudes upon their inner life that they seek to hide
- Emotionally indifferent individuals usually display a rigid personality and are unresponsive to subtle colours
- Each colour has its own significance; generally dark colours show depression and melancholy
- Bright colours show gaiety and comedy

Eliminate Allergy Technique (EAT)

Introduction to EAT

While the majority of allergy treatments for foods involve restricting foods, the Eliminate Allergy Technique (EAT) allows you to eat. There are 2 definitions of allergies often used: one, the **narrow** definition states that an allergy is an inappropriate **immune response** to an allergen, which could apply to anything from ragweed to nuts. Second, the **broad** definition of an allergy is an inappropriate **functional response** to an allergen causing fatigue, headaches, joint pain or abdominal discomfort. The Eliminate Allergy Technique addresses both definitions and eliminates allergies. Whether you do or do not have the typical "allergy" symptoms like a runny nose, itchy red watery eyes, coughing and wheezing, the EAT treatments will also help you to properly absorb vitamins, minerals, proteins, fats and sugars. Without proper absorption it is impossible to achieve optimal health. Unfortunately, many people taking supplements for iron, vitamin D or B12 deficiencies, as an example, may not see significant improvements because the problem truly lies in their ability to absorb the nutrient properly. There is no benefit if you cannot absorb it. By improving your absorption, food and environmental sensitivities can be effectively eliminated with EAT treatments. For example, vitamin A is crucial to mucous membranes. Without proper absorption your cells cannot defend themselves against airborne irritants, foods, microorganisms and chemicals. An EAT treatment for vitamin A will therefore strengthen the integrity of your cells to defend and protect themselves against external irritants, no longer triggering an immune response. Anyone suffering from symptoms of headaches, fatigue, bloating, gas, heartburn, arthritis, asthma or eczema are more likely to have food sensitivities including grains (wheat and gluten), dairy, nuts, corn, coffee, sugar, food additives, chocolate and alcohol.

How was EATs Discovered?

EAT is an enhancement of a treatment developed by Dr. Devi Nambudripad in 1983. She grew up with severe allergic symptoms including juvenile arthritis, eczema, indigestion, asthma and chronic fatigue. Her condition initially led to the study of nursing, where the common medical treatment was to avoid reaction causing foods and to take antihistamines or other pharmaceuticals. Dr. Nambudripad appeared to react to everything she consumed. She even reacted to all medications, except for Aspirin which she often used to make it through the day. The best treatment was to avoid more and more food. Unsatisfied, Dr. Nambudripad decided to study Chiropractic Medicine where she learned about Applied Kinesiology (muscle testing) and its application to food allergies. After comprehensive testing, it was concluded that she could only tolerate white rice and broccoli. The pain and symptoms subsided when her diet was limited to only these two foods. Dr. Nambudripad was able to maintain this diet for over 3 years! While studying acupuncture and Chinese Medicine, she found that acupuncture relieved symptoms caused by consuming an allergic food. The relief, unfortunately, was never permanent. One day while making dinner for her family she absent-mindedly ate a carrot, immediately bringing on symptoms of severe exhaustion. Her husband, an acupuncturist, gave her an acupuncture treatment right there on the kitchen table. After falling asleep she awoke feeling great and interestingly now able to tolerate carrots! This had never happened before. So what was different? During this treatment, a piece of carrot had been stuck to her arm. Dr. Nambudripad immediately started experimenting with holding onto various foods, vitamins, and minerals while receiving the acupuncture treatment. The knowledge she attained became the foundation of NAET (Nambudripad Allergy Elimination Technique) and ultimately the adaptation of EAT. NaturoMedic.com's EAT differs from Nambudripad's NAET because we utilize homeopathics instead of requiring a 24-hour avoidance period of the food or nutrient. We also teach a specific breathing technique to increase the treatment's effectiveness.

How do EATs Work?

EATs target the body's Autonomic Nervous System (ANS). The ANS helps your body function on autopilot so you do not have to think about things such as breathing, regulating your blood pressure and digesting food. The ANS has two parts: the parasympathetic nervous system and the sympathetic nervous system. The sympathetic nervous system is the body's accelerator; it speeds everything up. Breathing, blood flow to the muscles and heart rate all increase with sympathetic stimulation. It is commonly known as the "fight or flight" response directing you to run from (flight) or deal with (fight) a threat to your survival. The parasympathetic nervous system puts on the brakes. It slows everything down and allows your body to repair itself and digest food. Normally there is a balance between the two. During the treatment, we use alternating breathing patterns to stimulate both parts of the ANS. Deep breathing initiates the parasympathetic system and panting the sympathetic. We simultaneously apply pressure to acupuncture points on your back that correlate to your organs, known as the back shu points. These points run on either side of the spine, where all the nerves of the ANS leave the spine cord. By combining acupressure and breathing, we can reset the ANS, decrease allergies, promote absorption and encourage assimilation of nutrients for healing.

How do we know what to treat?

If necessary, blood work can be performed by your Allergist (or by NaturoMedic.com) to determine the foods that provoke an immune response or we can employ muscle testing. We use muscle testing to determine functional and energetic reactions to nutrients, foods or other allergens that the body cannot absorb or tolerate. Muscle testing assesses a functional response and not necessarily an immune response because we measure subtle frequencies of electromagnetic fields (EMF) in your body via your ANS. A weak muscle response indicates your body's ANS is rejecting or repelling the EMF of the substance you are holding. A strong muscle response indicates your body's ANS is accepting or attracting the EMF of the substance you are holding. In this way we can functionally assess which substances your body is reacting to. For example, while holding a vial of eggs, your body may give a strong muscle response suggesting that you are accepting of eggs. Alternatively, a weak muscle response indicates that your body is essentially having a negative functional reaction to eggs. At NaturoMedic.com, we implement the EAT technique to treat you for the substance, eventually leading to the desired strong muscle response thereby promoting absorption and encouraging assimilation of nutrients for healing.

What improvements will I see after getting EATs?

Most people experience slow incremental changes as the treatments progress. You might notice increased colour in the face, reduction of dark circles under the eyes, or stronger healthier nails and hair. We have also witnessed some dramatic changes. A seven year old boy presented with a severe allergy to peanuts, developing swelling and closing of the throat (anaphylaxis) when coming into contact with peanuts. After a series of EAT treatments, he was found to be completely clear of the allergy upon retesting at McMaster Children's Hospital. Another woman attended a lecture on EATs and allergies where Dr. Prytula demonstrated a treatment on eggs for her. She neglected to mention that she had anaphylactic reactions to eggs and went home to suffer greatly for the next few days as her body processed the treatment. She later reported to Dr. Prytula that, to her delight, she could now eat eggs without a problem and her overall health had greatly improved! After a series of EAT treatments, one gentleman suffering from shellfish anaphylaxis unknowingly ate some shellfish in a sauce without realizing it until finishing the meal. We have witnessed the resolution of many anaphylactic allergic conditions due to the EAT treatment.

Possible EAT Reactions

Is there a "normal" reaction after a successful EAT treatment? Some patients do not experience any change following their first EAT treatment. A few find the change to be very subtle and others may experience one or more symptoms from the list below. Anything you notice, other than being pain-free, with an overall sense of well-being mentally and physically, is a reaction. The intensity of the reaction(s) depends on many factors, such as the duration of the illness, the intensity of the illness and the status of the immune system. In most cases, if a reaction occurs, it will only last for a short period of time.

Possible Short-term Physical Reactions

- High/low energy, general body aches, temperature variations, extreme fatigue, sleepiness, insomnia, restlessness
- Tingling, twitching or pinprick sensation anywhere in the body, shooting to dull pain
- Headaches, ringing in the ears, blurred vision, sensations of hair like particles in the eye and numbness, choking, throat constriction
- Sneezing, coughing, tearing, post nasal drip, sensation of the dust-like particles in the lungs
- Increased blood pressure, palpitation, tightness in the chest, cardiac arrhythmia, decreased or increased heart rates, paroxysmal tachycardia, sudden venous congestion or varicose vein
- Abdominal bloating, nausea, belching, hiccups, hyperacidity, diarrhea, constipation
- Excessive or low libido
- A reoccurrence of old symptoms

Possible Short-term Emotional Reactions

- Anxiety, nervousness, depression, mood swings, fear, crying spells, butterfly sensation in the stomach, obsession, exacerbation of suicidal thoughts, laughing spells
- Cravings: salt, sugar, spices, sour things, coffee, popcorn, sweet smells (flower or perfumes), chemical smell (bleach), smell of sweat, etc.

Please note any symptoms you experience.

Emotional Allergy and/or Sensitivity

The origin of physical symptoms can often be traced back to an unresolved emotional trauma. For example, one patient's EAT treatments were continuously not holding. Upon investigation it was discovered that growing up her parents would have an intense argument at each meal. After an MRT session to resolve the emotional trauma around eating in a safe environment, the EAT treatments held.

Following a successful treatment for an allergen, the physical and nutritional allergy or sensitivity may never return. However the emotional allergy or sensitivity can return if you are not careful to avoid unpleasant things while eating or cooking. It is very important to respect food preparation and consumption for better assimilation of the nutrients and to avoid the recurrence of emotional allergies or sensitivities.

Develop Good Eating Habits and Prevent Emotional Blockages

Avoid eating when under stress and always try to have pleasant thoughts while eating. Positive thoughts will help with nutrient absorption; so enjoy your food. You can play your favorite music while you eat.

Many cultures bless their food before they eat, giving one a chance to clear the mind of all troubled emotions. Calming the mind before you eat helps to avoid digestive difficulties. Try to eat with people who share positive thoughts and make eating a pleasant event.

Diet: EAT patients are encouraged to eat non-allergic and non-sensitive food whenever possible and drink 5-8 glasses of clear, filtered water a day.

Exercise: Regular exercise is very important to the distribution of nutrients evenly in the body and stimulates the proper flow of energy along acupuncture meridians. Begin very slowly if you are very sick or have not exercised recently. It is also advisable to drink a large glass of water after exercising to help eliminate the toxins produced from the workout.

To EAT or Not To EAT? – That is the Question

EAT treatments may appear simple but they have a large impact. Energetic changes along the various meridians are taking place during and after the treatments. Food can help replenish your energy, so fasting is not recommended.

Eating Refined Food

Refined foods should be avoided. Eat more non-allergenic complex carbohydrates, fresh fruits and vegetables. In the initial stage, cook food well if it is hard to digest. If you are not a vegetarian, eat unprocessed lean meats. Avoid excess fat consumption, as these types of foods will slow down the energy circulation through the energy meridians.

Food Craving During Treatment

Most of the time, when you are treated for an allergen sensitivity with EAT, you may experience an unusual craving for that particular item or you may experience withdrawal symptoms. The reason for this is because the long-term allergy or sensitivity has created a huge deficiency of essential nutrients. The brain is simply demanding more essential nutrients for the body.

References:
1. Winning the War Against Asthma And Allergies or sensitivities or sensitivities, by Ellen W. Culter, ISBN 0-8273-8622-2
2. Say Goodbye to Illness, by Devi S. Nambudripad, ISBN 0-9658242-1-7

High Protein Diet & Insulin Resistance

The high protein diet is a weight loss program designed to help you lose fat but maintain your muscle mass. For a relatively short period of time the amount of carbohydrates (sugars and starches) and fats consumed are drastically reduced. The amount of protein however is supplemented to meet the body's daily requirements. Foods like breads, fruits, dairy, nuts and alcohol are restricted while low starch vegetables and leafy greens are increased. This is for the specific purpose of forcing your body to burn fat as well as correcting hormone imbalances that cause weight gain.

Sugars and starches are avoided for a number of reasons. Sugar is the body's main source of energy. As long as you feed your body sugar, it is more than happy to leave your fat stores alone making weight loss difficult. Additionally, sugars and starches raise the body's insulin levels. Over eating these foods triggers a hormone imbalance called insulin resistance. Insulin is the hormone secreted by the pancreas that helps regulate blood sugar. Insulin is required to help get the sugar from your blood into the body's cells where it is used to make energy. With excess sugar consumption, over time your pancreas becomes dysfunctional as a result of a sugar-rich diet, secreting more insulin than the body needs. This excessive insulin output will cause a number of health problems including weight gain (especially around the belly), high blood pressure and high cholesterol. Eventually cells will start to ignore the excess insulin and become insulin resistant. The pancreas releases more insulin to achieve the same goal of getting sugar into the cells. As the pancreas becomes fatigued, the blood sugar remains permanently high (type II diabetes).

The goal of the high protein diet is to lower insulin levels to such a degree that your pancreas is allowed to heal while your cells become sensitive to insulin again. Your pancreas is reset and the problems caused by excess insulin are reversed.

The plan is designed to achieve this over several stages:

- In the first stage, a person consumes supplemental protein throughout the day along with low carbohydrate vegetables, small amounts of low glycemic fruit and dairy (or alternatives), and a serving of meat. This phase lasts a minimum of 2 weeks or until the point at which most of the desired weight loss has occurred.
- The second stage slowly allows for the slow reintroduction of meat into the diet and takes away some supplemental protein.
- Stage three retrains the pancreas. Every day for the next two weeks, eating a full breakfast each morning will cause insulin to spike early in the day and remain low for the rest of the day.

- The final stage is a healthy lifestyle plan including all food groups.

The intention is to not to continue with protein supplements when you have reached your intended weight. The final goal is meant to be a reasonable lifestyle food plan to follow for life. The program is not a permanent cure for insulin resistance if you continue to eat high starch/sugar foods in excess after completing the first three stages. The pancreas can become dysfunctional again and the weight can be regained. If you are having trouble following the lifestyle plan, there may be other factors to take into consideration such as emotional eating, food sensitivities, unsuccessful habits and chronic infections to name a few.

Reference:
1. Chanh, T.T. The No-hassle Protein Diet Guide: The Unbalanced Diet Approach to a Slimmer You. 2000. Published by Ideal Protein.

Homeopathy

The extraordinary science of homeopathy emerged early in the 19th century. This well described system of medicine is now the second most used system in the world and its growth throughout the past 200 years has been rather extraordinary, especially in North America.

The founder, Dr. Samuel Hahnemann, began experimenting with the potential of homeopathy shortly after graduating from medical school. At the time (mid 1700s), the common medical practices of purging, bloodletting and administering toxic chemicals left him quite disillusioned and unsettled. His investigations brought forth the fundamental Principle of Similarity "like cures like" which states that a given substance can cure the same symptoms in a diseased person that it produces in a healthy person. For example, in 400 BC Hippocrates prescribed mandrake root to treat mania which incidentally was known to cause mania in a healthy person. In homeopathy, highly diluted substances are selected to treat health conditions based on the same set of symptoms produced when the crude form of that product is consumed by a healthy person. Take the example of a person presenting with insomnia associated with a racing mind and uncontrollable thoughts. Homeopathic *coffea* would typically be prescribed. Coffee consumed in excess is well-known to cause these symptoms, yet as a homeopathic preparation these are the symptoms it cures. This concept is not unfamiliar to the medical profession although it is not used in the same capacity. In 1983, a study in the New England Journal of Medicine reported that vitamin B6 can treat nerve damage but can also cause nerve damage in large doses.

Dr. Hahnemann continued to refine his philosophy to establish a highly systematized method of medical therapeutics that provide gentle solutions, by stimulating the body's own natural healing powers. From the late 1700s and into the 1800s, the effectiveness of homeopathy continued to grow, gaining most of its early popularity in the treatment of acute and epidemic disease throughout the world. During the cholera epidemic in the 1830s, the mortality rate for patients of homeopathy ranged from 2.4% to 21.1% while the rate for conventional medical care was over 50%. The first homeopathic hospital was opened in 1832 and subsequently homeopathic medical schools opened all over North America. By the early 1900s, there were 22 homeopathic medical schools in the United States, 100 homeopathic hospitals and over 1,000 homeopathic pharmacies. Boston University, Stanford University, University of Michigan, University of Iowa and New York Medical College were all institutions that taught homeopathy. Many well respected members of society were strong advocates of homeopathy including Henry Wadsworth Longfellow, Nathanial Hawthorne, Daniel Webster,

Louisa May Alcott, John D. Rockefeller, Charles Dickens, W.B. Yeats and Pope Pius X. Britain's Royal Family have been dedicated patrons since the early 1830s.

The success of homeopathy in treating infectious epidemic diseases contributed immensely to its popularity. Mortality (death) rates in homeopathic hospitals were often 50% to 88% less than those in medical hospitals. Only 3% of the 1,116 homeopathic patients of Cinncinati died during the 1849 cholera epidemic, as opposed to 48-60% of medical patients. The statistics for the yellow fever epidemic of 1878 showed 7.7% mortality for homeopathy patients in New Orleans and 16% for patients of conventional medical practitioners. The American Medical Association journal later estimated that allopathic mortality rates were actually 20-25%.

Homeopathic care was effective for a variety of acute and chronic illnesses. Patients had longer lives, prompting insurance companies to offer a 10% discount to homeopathic patients. The London Life Assurance Office announced in 1865 that "…persons treated by the homeopathic system enjoy more robust health, are less frequently attacked by disease and recover more steadily…medicines prescribed by homeopaths do not injure the constitution, whereas those employed by allopathists not unfrequently entail the most serious, and in many instances, fatal, consequences". Homeopathic life insurance companies were also being created. In 1870 the Homeopathic Manual Life Office of New York reported selling 7,927 policies to homeopathic advocates and 2,258 to non-homeopathic patients in less than 10 years. Of the two categories there had been 84 deaths (1%) in the first and 66 (3%) in second, further justifying the lower premiums offered to homeopathic patients.

At the beginning of World War I in 1914, 300 homeopathic physicians had commissions in the National Guard or regular army. By the end of the war in 1918, 1,862 homeopathic physicians had received commissions. Unfortunately, a decline in practice of homeopathy occurred in connection with new regulations from the American Medical Association and a decline in funding. The Flexner Report of 1910, released in Canada and the US enforced higher admission and graduation standards for medical schools. In addition, a strict adherence to mainstream science was required in their teaching. According to the report, too many doctors were being trained and too many medical schools existed. As a repercussion, many schools either amalgamated or closed and females were restricted from admission. Only graduates of these schools were permitted to write the medical licensing exams. Of the 20 homeopathic colleges in 1900, only 2 remained by 1923.

Today, homeopathic resurgence has become more apparent with nearly all French pharmacies selling homeopathic remedies and medicines. Homeopathy has a particularly strong following in Russia, India, Switzerland, Mexico, Germany, Netherlands, Italy, England and South America. Homeopathy has maintained a consistent tradition throughout the world. For example, homeopathic hospitals and outpatient clinics are part of England's national health system. There are over 120 homeopathic medical schools in India with four and five year programs. An article in the World Health Forum stated that "in the Indian subcontinent the legal position of the practitioners of homeopathy has been elevated to a professional level similar to that of a medical practitioner".

Homeopathy has been experiencing resurgence since the 1970s. The F.D.A. Consumer magazine reported a 1000% increase in homeopathic medical sales from the late 1970s to the early 1980s. The Western Journal of Medicine observed that patients of homeopathy tend to be better educated than the average citizen. Despite the oppression from the medical profession, homeopathy has survived. Mark Twain's eloquent words in 1890 continue to hold meaning today "The introduction of homeopathy forced the old school doctor to stir around and learn something of a rational nature about his business... You may honestly feel grateful that homeopathy survived the attempts of the allopathists (orthodox physicians) to destroy it".

Homeopathy is a remarkable therapy. Its non-invasive capability of stimulating the body's inherent defense and self-regulatory mechanisms is significantly effective. In homeopathy, disease is believed to arise from a weakness in a patient's defense mechanisms. It is a way in which our regulatory process can express what is happening inside the body, in response to multiple forms of stress. Homeopathics, derived from plants, minerals or chemical substances, attempt to maintain homeostasis. Homeopathy works in cooperation with the body's regulatory functions.

Homeopathy is a complex system of medicine. At NaturoMedic.com, we prescribe homeopathics on an individual basis to ensure that the appropriate substance is given. We seek to prescribe those that incorporate all your symptoms and will help your body to repair its defenses.

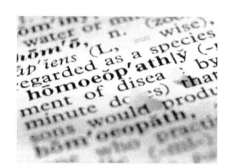

References:

1. Pizzorno & Murray. Textbook of Natural Medicine. 3rd ed. Vol. I. Churchill Livingstone. 2006.
2. Trattler, Better Health Through Natural Healing. McGraw-Hill, 1985.
3. http://www.wholehealthnow.com/homeopathy_info/history.html
4. http://www.homeopathic.com/Articles/Introduction_to_Homeopathy/A_Condensed_History_of_Homeopathy.html
5. Beck, Andrew H. (5). The Flexner report and the standardization of American medical education. The Journal of the American Medical Association. 2004. 291(17): 2139-40.
6. Coulter, H. Divided Legacy: the conflict between homeopathy and the American medical association. 1973. 2nd edition. North Atlantic Books. Berkeley, CA.
7. World Health Organization (WHO). Legal Status of Traditional Medicine and Complementary/Alternative Medicine: A Worldwide Review. 2001. http://apps.who.int/medicinedocs/pdf/h2943e/h2943e.pdf

Intravenous Myers Cocktail

The idea of receiving vitamins intravenously may seem strange and somewhat extreme. Are not IVs just for really sick people in the hospital? IV therapy can have significant health benefits for all of us. Let us answer some of your questions. What is a Myers? Why do I need it? What is it good for? What are the dangers?

What is an IV Myers?

This treatment is a modification of an IV vitamin and mineral formula used by the late John Myers, MD. He was a physician from Baltimore, Maryland and a pioneer in the use of IV vitamins and minerals. As part of the overall treatment of various medical problems this modified IV consists of vitamins and minerals in differing proportions depending on the patient's condition.

Why do I need it?

You may be fighting a cold or flu bug, stressed, run down or fatigued. The treatment can also be administered prior to an upcoming stressful situation to help you cope more easily. If you have been fighting a cold all season or your energy is low, these symptoms are signs that the body is not balanced. It is a reflection that the body is not healthy.

Our body is powered by trillions of cells which are fueled by nutrients in our food. During times of ill health, the cells need nutrients to get the job done. More importantly, we need to get the nutrients into the cells where they can be efficiently used. If nutrients remain outside the cells, the kidneys and liver will filter them out. Nutrients gain entry into the cells in two ways. First, by absorption, where nutrients slip through the cell wall (membrane). Secondly, by actively being transported across the cell wall (membrane). This requires energy. When cells are sick, they are not able to perform their functions correctly, such as actively transporting the nutrients into the cell. This problem is bypassed by forcing the nutrients into the cell through absorption. When given in high concentration, intravenous nutrients enter the cell by sheer force of numbers.

Could I just take it orally?

There is nothing wrong with taking supplements orally. However during times of ill health, the body needs more nutrients and the absorption of these nutrients may be compromised. When taking supplements orally, we are limited by a few factors, as nutrients in the supplements need to get from the stomach and into the bloodstream. Appropriate digestive enzymes and hydrochloric acid must be present in order to break down the supplement. As we get older, the natural production of hydrochloric acid and enzymes is reduced. From the stomach, the supplement travels to the small and large intestines where absorption occurs and it enters the bloodstream, then the cells. By the time the nutrient has finally reached the bloodstream, approximately 70% has been lost in transit. Another factor that needs to be considered is that the body has a saturation point. This means anything above and beyond a certain point the body will not be able to absorb. A good example is with vitamin C. The average individual will be able to take approximately 1000 mg with no ill effects. However, if one increases oral vitamin C consumption to 5000-30,000 mg, the body's saturation point will be met and the rest will be expelled through a bowel movement, possibly diarrhea. However, intravenous and intramuscular administration produces an immediate and significant increase in concentration because it is delivered right into the bloodstream bypassing the stomach and allowing us to increase the amount of nutrients significantly. We administer approximately 2,500-5,000mg of vitamin C. Other ingredients that support body function and the immune system included in the IV are magnesium, B1, B5, B complex, B12, B6, calcium and various minerals.

Who will benefit?

Meyers cocktails have been administered to treat acute asthma, migraines, fatigue, chronic fatigue syndrome, fibromyalgia, colds and flu's, upper respiratory tract infections, chronic sinusitis and seasonal allergies. One of the major nutrients included is vitamin C. Vitamin C is crucial for the immune system, which is made up of white blood cells. The levels of vitamin C in the blood achieved by the IV will enhance the activity of the white blood cells or, in essence, enhance and stimulate the immune system. The immune system utilizes the vitamin C to fight viral and bacterial infections (*E.coli, Staphylococcus aureus, Pseudomonas aeruginosa, etc*). It can aid in preventing diabetes and its complications, asthma and other allergy related conditions. It enables the body to better deal with environmental pollution and toxic chemicals and inhibits the formation of cancer-causing compounds in the body. All of these benefits can be achieved just from vitamin C, not including the many benefits of the other nutrients and in sixty minutes!

What are the dangers?

Since we are administering these nutrients intravenously there are some precautions that must be taken into consideration. First and foremost, patients must eat before receiving an IV. The concentration of vitamins and minerals in the IV will reduce blood sugar levels. If the patient has not eaten adequately they may find themselves dizzy and light headed and may even pass out. Also, due to the concentration of the vitamins and minerals in the IV, the patient may feel a dull ache above the IV site.

How long does it take?

Barring any of the above instances, the whole procedure takes sixty minutes. When first administered, a slower rate is given. The number of treatments needed is dependent upon the patient's condition. If the patient has a severe cold or flu, one or more successive therapy sessions will be needed to attain optimal health. Some patients utilize this therapy for prevention and will get a treatment on a monthly basis or more frequently if necessary.

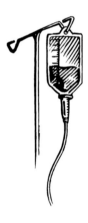

Intravenous Vitamin C and Cancer

Benefits of the IV Administration of Vitamin C

- IV route is the only route to acquire therapeutic concentration.

- IV vitamin C stops proliferation of cancer cells by inhibiting the enzyme hyaluronidase which cancer cells emit to break down and invade healthy tissues.

- IV vitamin C supports the immune system, assists in the healing of wounds and protects against infection.

- IV vitamin C is preferentially toxic to cancer cells by increasing intracellular hydrogen peroxide. Cancer cells cannot process the hydrogen peroxide due to a lack of the enzyme catalase, which normal cells have in abundance.

- IV vitamin C corrects an ascorbate deficiency, often seen in cancer patients.

- IV vitamin C helps prevent cellular free radical damage.

- IV vitamin C increases the quality of life.

- IV vitamin C extends life.

- IV vitamin C works alongside chemotherapy.

- According to the National Cancer Institute, 1990, Dr. Donald Henson summarized a NCI Symposium on vitamin C: "The take home message was that vitamin C has multiple complex effects on a variety of biological activities, perhaps wider than any other nutrient. Many of these effects seem related to its chemical properties and not to its role as a vitamin."

Vitamin C's Effects on Killing Cancer

In the book Cancer and Vitamin C by Cameron and Pauling, a Canadian physician, Dr. W.J. McCormick, hypothesized in 1954 and 1959 that cancer is a disease associated with a deficiency in vitamin C. He recognized that the changes in tissues from scurvy are identical to the alterations of invading cancer cells. Dr. McCormick surmised that since this nutrient (vitamin C) is capable of preventing damage from scurvy, then it may have similar effects in cancer. The evidence that cancer patients are found to almost invariably be depleted of vitamin C supported this view.

Cameron and Pauling also state, "Most important of all, we are led to the conclusion that the administration of this harmless substance, ascorbic acid (vitamin C), might provide us with an effective means of permanently suppressing neoplastic cellular proliferation and invasiveness, in other words an effective means of controlling cancer. Ascorbic acid (vitamin C) in adequate doses might prove to be the ideal cytostatic agent."

According to the 4th Quarter, 2000 Journal of Orthomolecular Medicine, Riordan, Riordan & Casciari concluded from their research, "vitamin C is toxic to tumor cells. Concentrations of vitamin C that kill tumor cells can be achieved in humans using intravenous vitamin C infusions."

One study reported in the Journal of Nutrition and Biochemistry in July 2006, concluded that the combined treatment with retinoic acid (vitamin A) and ascorbic acid (vitamin C) inhibited the proliferation of human breast cancer cells. The combination altered the gene expression of antioxidation processes as well as the proliferation inhibitory pathway.

In 1991, the Journal of Oncology reported two cases of complete cancer regression in response to high-dose ascorbic acid therapy.

Vitamin C's Effects on Quality and Duration of Life

According to a study reported in the Canadian Medical Association Journal in March 2006, early clinical research showed that high-dose vitamin C, given by intravenous and oral routes, may improve symptoms and prolong life in patients with terminal cancer. The study found three well-documented cases of advanced cancer where patients had unexpectedly long survival times after receiving high-dose intravenous vitamin C therapy.

In a trial of vitamin C in the Vale of Leven Hospital, researchers described the quite dramatic relief of bone pain in four out of five patients with expanding skeletal metastases. Of equal importance was the observation that most of the ascorbate-treated patients entered a period of increased well-being and general improvement. In another clinical report in the same trial, 50 patients with advanced cancer received 10g of vitamin C or more per day. It was expected that most of these patients (90%) would die within about three months. In fact, only half of them had died on or before the 100th day after being deemed to be "untreatable" at the time the administration of ascorbate was begun. In similar trials, 100 ascorbate-treated patients have lived on average about 300 days longer than their matched controls. In addition, it is the researchers' strong clinical impression that they have lived happier lives during this terminal period.

In another study published by the Journal of Korean Medical Sciences in February 2007, terminal cancer patients reported significantly higher scores for physical, emotional and cognitive function after administration of vitamin C. In symptom scale, the patients reported significantly lower scores for fatigue, nausea/vomiting, pain and appetite loss after the administration of vitamin C.

Vitamin C's Positive Interaction with Chemotherapy and Radiation

A study published in March-April 2007 from the journal of Alternative Therapies in Health and Medicine, concluded that non-prescription antioxidants and other nutrients do not interfere with therapeutic modalities (chemotherapy and radiation) for cancer. The meta-analysis found consistent results since 1970 from 280 peer-reviewed in vitro and in vivo studies. Including 50 human studies involving 8,521 patients, from which 5,081 were given nutrients. Furthermore, the supplements enhanced the killing therapeutic modalities (chemotherapy and radiation) for cancer, decreased their side effects and protected normal tissue. In 15 of the human studies, the 3,738 patients who took non-prescription antioxidants and other nutrients actually had increased survival.

In a review paper in The Journal of American Nutraceutical Association, Block & Evans reviewed all English articles listed in Index Medicus between the years 1990-2000 related to antioxidant and interactions with anticancer drugs or radiation and concluded that "there is a rational basis for the continued use of antioxidant agents as a therapeutic adjunct in cancer therapy."

Another study published in the Journal of Chemotherapy in October 2005 indicated that vitamin C enhances the antitumor activity of two chemotherapeutic drugs and sensitizes cancer cells to drug-induced cell death. The data suggested that vitamin C supplementation may improve the efficacy of chemotherapy for esophageal cancer. Yet another study reported in the medical journal Cancer Treatment Review in March 2007 concluded that none of the trials reported evidence of significant decreases in efficacy from antioxidant supplementation during chemotherapy. Many of the studies indicated that antioxidant supplementation resulted in either increased survival times, increased tumor responses, or both, as well as fewer toxicities than controls.

For more information on vitamin C and cancer please refer to our blog at www.NaturoMedic.com.

Additional reading:

1. Um, M. The benefits of IV vitamin C: a treatment for cancer. May 2008. http://www.naturomedic.com/Portals/168760/docs/IV-Vitamin-C2.pdf
2. Prytula, M. Intravenous vitamin C in cancer management. Feb 2008. http://www.naturomedic.com/Portals/168760/docs/IV-C-Prytula1.pdf

References:

1. Cameron E and Pauling L. Cancer and Vitamin C. Philadelphia, PA: Camino Books 1993.

2. Padayatty SJ, Riordan HD, Hewitt SM, Katz A, Hoffer LJ, Levine M. Intravenously administered vitamin C as cancer therapy: three cases. Canadian Medical Association Journal. 2006 Mar 28;174(7):956-7.

3. Padayatty SJ, Sun H, Wang Y, et al. Vitamin C pharmacokinetics: implications for oral and intravenous use. Ann Intern Med 2004;140:533-7.

4. Riordan NH, Riordan HD, Casciari JJ. Clinical and experimental experiences with intravenous vitamin C. Journal of Orthomolecular Medicine 2000;15:201-3.

5. Simone CB 2nd, Simone NL, Simone V, Simone CB. Antioxidants and other nutrients do not interfere with chemotherapy or radiation therapy and can increase kill and increase survival, Part 2. Alternative Therapies in Health and Medicine. 2007 Mar-Apr;13(2):40-7.

6. Block KI, Koch AC, Mead MN, Tothy PK, Newman RA, Gyllenhaal C. Impact of antioxidant supplementation on chemotherapeutic efficacy: a systematic review of the evidence from randomized controlled trials. Cancer Treatment Review. 2007 Aug;33(5):407-18.

7. Yeom CH, Jung GC, Song KJ. Changes of terminal cancer patients health-related quality of life after high dose vitamin C administration. Journal of Korean Medical Science. 2007 Feb;22(1):7-11.

Manipulation

Manipulation is a manual maneuver used to restore maximal, pain-free movement of the muscular skeletal system. The history of manipulation of the spine and extremities begins as early as Hippocrates in 640 BC. There is evidence throughout Asia and India that there is a possibility of earlier roots. In China, a distinct branch of Traditional Chinese Medicine called Tui Na, was devoted to manipulative techniques that date back to 2700 BC. Naturopathy and Chiropractic care were taught in the same colleges up until the 1950s. Manipulation techniques were considered part of the naturopathic education. Today these two schools of thought are no longer in the same building. Manipulation is still a strong part of the naturopathic curriculum and remains a requirement for graduation and licensure for Naturopathic Medicine.

Manipulation adjusts bones to increase mobility and correct misalignment. Naturopathic manipulation focuses on both soft tissue and bone alignment similar to a chiropractic adjustment. These techniques use a high-velocity thrust to achieve joint cavitation (popping noise). This form of manipulation differs from other forms of manipulation which incorporate stretching, pressure and mobilization to correct the alignment of the spine and organs. Other forms of manipulation may include lymphatic drainage and cranial sacral therapy involving subtle adjustments. Naturopaths use manipulation as part of their therapeutic regimen and do not rely on this technique as their sole method of treatment. We believe that misalignment could be the result of an underlying cause. For example, in acupuncture there are specific points that run along the spine and relate to internal organs, known as the Back-Shu points. A dysfunction in one of these organs could affect the musculoskeletal system and lead to a misalignment. Naturopathic treatment in this case would focus on improving the organ and secondarily addressing the spine.

The importance of manipulation as a therapy centers on the strong interrelationship between the spine and the structure and function of the body. An imbalance in the musculoskeletal system plays a role in health. It can lead to an interference with the nervous system and the body's ability to heal itself. The combination of the muscular and skeletal systems account for over half the body's mass and therefore use the most amount of energy. A decrease in function places more stress on other systems to give more energy to the musculoskeletal system. Muscles have the ability to pull bones out of alignment. If left unaddressed, the bones will remain misaligned which can lead to compensation from other muscles and the continuation of this cycle of applying pressure to more bones and joints. The resulting posture affects nerve function, increases pain, inflammation and general discomfort. By correcting the soft tissue and bones of the musculoskeletal system, naturopathic manipulation can improve the body's ability to rebalance the nervous system and create homeostasis in the body.

Manipulation techniques have come a long way since its early documentation, in which practitioners were often referred to as "bone breakers". The techniques have been refined to provide a gentler, high-velocity, low impact thrust to correct misalignments of the spine. At NaturoMedic.com, your ND is fully trained in naturopathic manipulation and is capable of using this therapy as an adjunctive treatment to your healing process. If you continually need to be adjusted there are

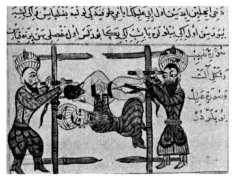

many reasons for this. You may want to read about Prolotherapy (for tendons & ligaments being stretched), Trigger Point Injections (for muscle spasms), Neural Therapy (for nerve irritations) or MRT (for subconscious emotions).

Manipulation during traction in medieval Turkey: Le Premier Manuscrit Chirurgical Turc de Charaf-Ed-Din (1465). (British Museum)
http://terapibekamkeiroprektik.blogspot.co m/2010/12/chiropractic-dalam-islam.html

Reference:
1.   Pizzorno & Murray. Textbook of Natural Medicine. 3rd ed. Vol. I. Churchill Livingstone. 2006.

Microorganism Elimination Technique (M.E.T.)

Microorganisms are a constant threat to our bodies, well-being, energy and vitality. Viruses, bacteria, mold and fungi can steal nutrients and force the body to use up resources to fight the infection and deal with the toxins released by the damaged infected tissue.

The M.E.T. or Microorganism Elimination Technique utilizes muscle testing or electrodermal testing, to detect the possible presence of specific pathogens/microorganisms. These foreign microbes may presently be the "causal factors" for compromised immune systems, preventing individuals from achieving optimal health.

This therapy helps to energetically identify the suspected microorganism(s) and direct the immune system to attack it. Once neutralized, the immune response is reset, preventing any further attack on the remaining healthy tissue.

How is M.E.T. Performed?
An M.E.T. session takes approximately 15 minutes to complete. The frequency of the treatments depends on the vitality of the individual, the severity of the pathology and the stealth capability of the microorganism.

The practitioner places a vial (containing the electromagnetic signature of a microorganism) in one hand and uses muscle testing on the other arm to evaluate the strength and weakness of the muscle. Once it is determined which microorganisms are possibly causing the body a problem, acupressure is then applied to attune the immune response to the electromagnetic dynamics of a specific microorganism.

A dietary adjustment of NO sugar or food with high sugar content is required for approximately 12 hours after the treatment.

What is a Microorganism?
A microorganism is a bacteria, parasite, virus, mold or fungus that contains an energetic signature or biological marker that the immune system identifies as foreign. This means it does not have the same markers as healthy cells. When foreign cells or materials are identified, the body sends signals to the immune system to attack the area where the foreign substance exists, waging a war. Joint pain in arthritis, for instance, can be as a result of the body identifying a microorganism as an invader and the immune system then wages war on that microorganism.

Regrettably, when this war takes place, the immune system will not only attack the foreign invader, it attacks the healthy tissues in that area as well. After this attack on the tissue, the body is weakened and left to repair the damage from the

255

attack. Unfortunately, this well-intentioned process may not actually destroy the microorganism. When under attack, some microorganisms with stealth capabilities retreat back into other tissues and other areas of the body, so that only a small amount of the foreign microbe could be eliminated. This process takes time, with each treatment it is similar to giving the scent to a hunting dog (immune system). After the microorganism is cleared, we then have to stop the immune system from waging war on other tissues by mistake.

Stealth Microorganisms

In chronic infections, the microorganism evades the immune system by several means. First of all it hides, typically in the areas of poor circulation (caused by heavy metals and chemicals). Secondly, the microorganism learns how to dominate the host's behaviour and immune system. Thirdly, the microorganism creates a better breeding ground for itself by producing peptides and other informational substances that create acidity and toxicity. This decreases the circulation lowering the temperature to benefit the microorganism and discouraging the immune system from accessing the infected area.

There are many other mechanisms that microorganisms use to maintain their stealth capability. Ultimately, a microorganism's primary goal is self-preservation. When western science cannot detect these microorganisms in infected tissues, the corresponding diseases are wrongly labeled as being autoimmune diseases. This is where the body attacks itself. In coronary heart disease and stroke, microorganisms have been identified as being the suspected cause. These include: *herpes viruses, chlamydia, h. pylori, strep, nanobacteria* and *salmonella*. In Multiple Sclerosis they have identified *herpes virus 6, mycoplasmas, borrelia* and *cytomegalovirus*. In osteoarthritis, they have identified *mycoplasmas* and *chlamydia*. In Parkinson's disease, *mycoplasmas, borrelia, chlamydia* and *herpes viruses*. In ALS or Lou Gerhig's disease, *mycoplasmas, borrelia, herpes simplex 1* and *2, cytomegalovirus* and *human herpes virus 6*. Cancer is often caused by a combination of numerous viruses, bacteria, fungi and parasites.

Toning Down the Immune System

After the stealth microorganism is eliminated, the immune system may still be sending continual attacks on the healthy tissues and the surrounding areas. Due to the stealth capability of the microorganism the immune system does not know when it has won the battle. This attack causes a breakdown of the healthy tissues. The repair of these tissues requires proper nutrition. Without proper nutrition, the body cannot effectively repair the damage and this attack can ultimately cause internal scaring and possibly chronic pain. M.E.T. puts a stop to the continuous attack on the healthy tissues after it has specifically pinpointed the foreign invader and destroyed it.

Note: If you have a severe pathology, continuing with the M.E.T. treatment is strongly recommended once the microorganism is gone. Otherwise you may experience severe pain due to the immune system's assault on healthy tissues.

How are Microorganisms treated?

Using muscle testing has allowed us to identify microbes possibly responsible for causing various disorders and diseases. The foundation of the treatment is to first alert the immune system, then to deactivate the microorganism and if necessary interrupt the pattern of pain sequences throughout the body. The process may need to isolate the different phases and levels of a microorganism in order to re-educate the autonomic system to most effectively repair damaged portions of the body.

Why Muscle Testing?

Muscle testing is used to energetically assess if an electromagnetic signature of a microorganism is involved in a health problem. From a strictly scientific perspective tissue biopsies, cultures and several other tests would need to be performed to locate a microorganism. Therefore this process could amount to hundreds, if not thousands of dollars in costs, not to mention irreparable damage done to the body due to the biopsy. Modern medicine cannot detect these microorganisms without very expensive lab tests. When we find a microorganism's electromagnetic signature, this does not mean you have an infection. It also does not mean that you do not. However, we have noticed that by clearing these electromagnetic signatures people's health significantly improves.

M.E.T. is used in Virtually any Disease for Patients of any Age

The more severe the pathology and the longer the pathology has persisted, the more treatments are needed. In addition to arthritis, M.E.T. can be used on medical diagnoses of Lupus, Fibromyalgia, early stages of M.S., Crohn's disease, colitis and autoimmune disorders. We have used it to treat cancer and heart diseases as well with variable results.

Other therapies that may need to be performed in conjunction with M.E.T. to kill stealth microorganisms include: IV ozone, chelation IV vitamins and minerals and E.A.T. The Eliminate Allergy Technique can electromagnetically reprogram the body to turn off extreme immune responses and then achieve maximum absorption of nutrients required to attain optimal health.

Other factors that may hinder the success of M.E.T. in getting results include: stress, weak or diseased organs, heavy metals, hormonal imbalance, drugs, chemicals, diet, food allergies, circulation, toxic emotions, subconscious emotions, weather conditions, environmental allergies and lack of exercise.

Mental Reprogramming Technique (M.R.T.)

Our Mental Reprograming Technique addresses the emotional component of disease, both functional and pathological, in a safe and effective physiological way. It is human nature to have an emotional response to significant events in our lives. Sometimes however, our bodies will hold onto a strong response that can eventually cause an imbalance in health. Less than 10% of thought is conscious. The remaining 90% is subconscious (unconscious). When we experience something that creates an emotional reaction, whether positive or negative, both our conscious and subconscious record it. Humans naturally follow the pleasure/pain principle, in which we avoid the negative and gravitate towards the positive. In our mind, our subconscious and conscious thoughts perceive threats and rewards to help reinforce pleasure stimulus and stay away from pain.

These mechanisms sometimes also create a physiological or pathological response to certain stimuli. For example, you may be having a conversation with a loved one and they make a comment with a certain body language or tone of voice attached to it. Your subconscious immediately responds. "I heard this before, I know how this goes". Inevitably an argument results. A salesperson could hit that emotional buy button in trying to get you to purchase something you do not really need. These automatic reactions are due to a previous emotional response that has been "locked" into your sympathetic nervous system. These responses are based on strong negative or positive emotions that have been attached to past events. In many instances you may not be aware of the conscious or subconscious emotion that manifests as a symptom of disease. Driving down the street, a car goes by with a sound similar to what happened in a previous accident. The subconscious, determined to ensure our survival, triggers the fight, flight or freeze alarm. This can cause one to cringe, have muscle spasms, headaches, anxiety, etc. The M.R.T attempts to delete the physiological subconscious and associated emotional response created in the body.

How does M.R.T. work?

The NaturoMedic.com ND uses muscle testing, body reflex points and semantic reactions (physiological reactions to memories or words) to assist and guide you to recall an emotional pattern, similar to a computer operator engaging a specific program. We work with you, assisting you to experience different thoughts and emotions (e.g. "I'm ok loving myself and my body" or "I'm ok forgiving myself" or "I'm ok forgiving that which has offended me"). During this process, your conscious thought scans your subconscious for other times where you may have seen, heard or felt the experience that led to the emotional impact. Remember the example of ladies saying "it is safe to lose weight" after using weight gain as emotional protection from the outside world (possibly from undue sexual attention). While you mentally hold the emotional memory, the NaturoMedic.com ND stimulates the associated acupressure points or pulse points to release the emotional intensity and delete the physiological response attached to it. The M.R.T. seeks to normalize a neurological imbalance by using a physical stimulus to break up the physical reaction to the emotion, allowing for a change in physiology. This can be so effective at removing past traumas, that when people attempt to recall the traumatic memory, they have difficulties. Some even recall the trauma as being a third party (once removed, like watching a movie) instead of first party (feeling it, being in the movie). They no longer experience it, but simply observe it.

Homeopathics and Western Botanicals can be used to help assist and reinforce the treatment.

Is M.R.T. treatment safe?

Yes. The NaturoMedic.com ND uses a safe and gentle stimulation of acupressure points. The entire procedure is not unpleasant and patients often express immediate relief following the point treatment.

Please note: M.R.T. treatment is NOT a substitute for psychological or psychiatric therapy. It will delete the trauma, however it will not teach you to not walk down the same street or not fall into the same hole. M.R.T. works in conjunction with psychotherapy and counseling. It may take 1 to 5 treatments to repair a strong emotional response.

What are emotions?

In the past, emotions were considered psychologically based. Scientific discoveries have however shown that emotions are physiologically based. According to the Longman Dictionary of Psychology and Psychiatry, emotions are "A complex reaction pattern of the changes in nervous, visceral and skeletal-muscle tissues response to a stimulus... As a strong feeling, emotion is usually directed towards a specific person or event and involves widespread physiological changes, such as increased heart rate and inhibition of peristalsis."

Furthermore, recent advancements in neuroscience demonstrate that emotions are an interaction between chains of amino acids, which form neuropeptides and receptors. Therefore, emotions are normal physiological (organic) processes in the body, some of which are pleasant and others which are not. When an emotional response is happening at an inappropriate time, it is producing abnormal physiology, illness symptoms and possibly contributing to pathology.

We feel different emotions in different parts of the body, in different ways. Ancient acupuncturists correlated the different emotions to different organ meridians in our body. For example, fear to the kidney, anger to the liver, grief to the lungs, etc. (*please refer to Chinese Herbal Patents for more information*)

Although the primary locations for the physiology of emotions are in the brain, spine, autonomic nervous system and acupuncture circuits, emotions do affect any and all parts of the body in a physiological way. Researchers have now demonstrated that emotional bio-chemicals travel to almost every cell in the body.

Who should use M.R.T.?
M.R.T. is for the individual in pursuit of excellent health, quality of life, inner joy and peace in coping with life's daily challenges and for the fulfillment of dreams and goals. M.R.T. is a powerful technique that allows for transition and transformation as it discharges old emotional-reality imprints. This procedure is done clearly, rapidly and thoroughly. As the physiological and nervous system attachments to the emotional response are cleared, they are removed from the subconscious and do not return unless they are re-imprinted by re-traumatization.

Ozone

Ozone is the active form of oxygen consisting of 3 atoms of oxygen instead of the usual two atoms. It is created by passing an electrical spark through a tube with medical grade oxygen. Another way ozone is created is by lightning during a thunderstorm. This creates the fresh smell we experience after a storm.

Is Ozone a New Therapy?

No. Ozone was discovered in 1840 in Germany by Christian Schonbein. Documentation of ozone therapy can be traced back to 1881 when Dr. Kellogg mentioned its use as a disinfectant the treatment of diphtheria. In 1885, the Florida Medical Association published "Ozone" by Dr. Charles J. Kenworthy, MD, detailing the use of ozone for therapeutic uses. Ozone was used by Benedict Lust, the father of naturopathic medicine. Since then, many more uses have been discovered for ozone. Today, after 125 years of usage, ozone therapy is a recognized modality in sixteen nations..

Is Ozone Harmful?

Ozone is an extremely powerful purifier. Interestingly, ozone is used in water treatment plants to sterilize equipment and neutralize chemicals. When we hear reports of a high ozone count, we know there is actually a high smog and pollution count. Unlike all of the different pollutants (nitric oxide, sulphuric oxide), ozone is easily measured and therefore the ozone count is used to tell how high the pollution is. When pollution is high, the earth creates ozone in an attempt to heal and purify itself, keeping our air breathable. Ozone is extremely beneficial when used properly.

Effects of Ozone:

- Kills bacteria
- Kills fungi
- Kills viruses
- Improves circulation
- Purifies and detoxifies
- Disinfects and sterilizes
- Promotes healing

Types of Ozone Treatments:

- Injection
- Intravenous Auto-hemotherapy
- Insufflation
- Ozonated water
- Ozonated olive oil
- Ozone with colonics

Diseases Treatable with Ozone

These include but are not limited to:

- Immunosuppressed diseases: AIDS, cancer and chronic viral diseases (such as hepatitis and herpes)
- Gangrenous conditions
- Circulatory conditions: atherosclerosis, stroke, senile dementia

261

- Gynecological infections: candida trichomonas and gardinerella
- Arthrosis (diseases of the joints)
- Osteoarthritis
- Burns, wounds and ulcers
- Macular degeneration

Intravenous Auto-hemotherapy/Direct IV
- Hepatitis B and C
- Herpes simplex
- Herpes zoster
- Lyme Disease

Topical Ozone
- Disinfectant and deodorizer (practiced during WWI)
- External ulcers
- Burns
- Skin lesions (wounds)
- Local infections (herpes simplex, herpes zoster)
- Eye injuries and infections

Rectal Insufflation
- Ulcerous colitis
- Anal fistulae and fissures
- Proctitis (stages I and II)
- Hepatitis B and C
- Immunomodulation (complementary in oncology)

References:
1. Renate Viebahn-Hänsler , Olga Sonia León Fernández & Ziad Fahmy (2012): Ozone in Medicine: The Low-Dose Ozone Concept—Guidelines and Treatment Strategies, Ozone: Science & Engineering: The Journal of the International Ozone Association, 34:6, 408-424. http://dx.doi.org/10.1080/01919512.2012.717847
2. Renate Viebahn-Hänsler. The use of ozone in medicine. 2002. 4th edition. Karl F. Haug publishers Heidelberg. Huegelsheim, Germany.

Prolotherapy

Regenerative Injection Therapy (RIT)

Prolotherapy is another name for Regenerative Injection Therapy (RIT). RIT is useful for addressing many different types of musculoskeletal pain. Demonstrated success has occurred with back pain, arthritis, fibromyalgia, unresolved whiplash injuries, sports injuries, carpal tunnel syndrome, partially torn tendons, ligaments and cartilage, chronic tendonitis, degenerated or herniated discs, TMJ and sciatica. RIT is a natural technique that stimulates the bodies healing mechanisms to repair the tendons and ligamentous structures underlying the painful area. Some physicians refer to RIT as spot welding for the joints.

What is Prolotherapy/RIT?

RIT is a highly effective, yet little known, method of treating chronic ligament and tendon weaknesses. Ligaments are the structural "connective tissue bands" that secure bones to bones. Ligaments can become weak from overuse or can become injured. With the blood supply to ligaments, tendons and bone being very limited, healing without prolotherapy is often slow, not always complete and the ligaments may not heal back to their original strength or endurance. Ligaments have many nerve endings including proprioceptors to show us where our joint is in space (i.e. whether it is bent or extended). There are also pain receptors that are present for our protection to share with us when tissues are getting close to or are being damaged. Tendons are the tissues which connect muscles to bones and tendons may also become injured and cause pain. When tendons and ligaments become strained or injured the joint no longer articulates properly resulting in pain, stiffness, inflammation, crepitus (cracking) and various levels of discomfort.

RIT works by stimulating localized precision inflammation. The basic premise of prolotherapy is that a substance (called a proliferant) is injected into the affected or weakened ligaments or tendons. The solution is usually made up of dextrose and normal saline. This leads to local inflammation which turns on the healing process. The growth of new ligament and tendon tissue is then stimulated. The ligament and tendon tissue which forms as a result of RIT is significantly thicker and stronger than normal tissue. This healing response occurs for up to 6 weeks but during the first week after the treatment the connective tissue fibers that form are quite small and may break when put under stress. So it is advisable not to exercise for the first week after treatment.

RIT is painful, but the pain from treatment is comparatively insignificant versus the everyday chronic pain experienced by the patient. For those who fear needles, as one patient so eloquently said "if I would have known it was going to be that many injections, I would have never done it". In the same breath "If I would have known it would give that much relief I would have done it a lot sooner". To assist patients with low pain tolerance the Naturopathic Doctor may give the patient topical freezing (cool spray), local anesthesia or homeopathy. Most patients receive the treatments without pain killers.

How many treatments?

Four to six treatments is the average for an area treated. Treatment response varies with each individual and the patients healing ability. Historical research suggests RIT should be performed every 2-6 weeks as most of the healing of ligaments occurs over a 2-6 week period. As healing progresses, the quantity of injections in volume and number required per treatment decreases. The pain will continue to diminish with each treatment.

You should continue your treatments until you are healed. After treatment commences, your response to therapy will give a more accurate estimate as to how many injections may be needed.

Are you a good candidate for RIT?

RIT strengthens specific areas, eliminating pain by stimulating the growth of healthy, strong new tissue by your body's own immune system.

What is the success rate with different joints?

We cross referenced research on prolotherapy for the feet, hands, knees, hips, low back, and shoulders to answer these questions.

I am too old, it will not work for me!

The average age for the studies conducted on the above joints is between 54 and 62.

How does this help my pain?

Average pain levels went from between 5.6-7 (10 being the worst) to between 2.3 - 2.9 after prolotherapy.

I have had this pain for a long time, it will not work for me.

Average years of pain included in these studies range from 4.5 to 5.3 years. 33-38% of participants were told no other treatment options were available.

My walking is compromised how much can my walking improve?

For patients with:

- Foot conditions, 37% before prolotherapy were either wheel chair bound, used a cane or walker or could walk less than 3 blocks. After prolotherapy, only 5% were so compromised. 32% were now able to walk more than 3 blocks. Another 32% were able to walk without restriction after the treatment.

- Knee issues, 42% before prolotherapy were either wheel chair bound, used a cane or walker or could walk less than 3 blocks. After prolotherapy, only 9% were so compromised. 33% were now able to walk more than 3 blocks. Another 65% were able to walk without restriction after the treatment.
- Low back, 32% before prolotherapy were either wheel chair bound, used a cane or walker or could walk less than 3 blocks. After prolotherapy, only 5% were so compromised. 27% were now able to walk more than 3 blocks. Another 21% were able to walk without restriction after the treatment.
- Hip issues, 27% before prolotherapy were either wheel chair bound, used a cane or walker or could walk less than 1 block. After prolotherapy, all participants were now able to walk more than 1 block. Another 20% were able to walk without restriction after the treatment.

I want to get back into sports!
Athletic ability went from:

- Foot issues, 42% of participants could perform athletics for less than 10 minutes prior to prolotherapy. Only 5% could after. Another 11% were able to exercise without restriction.
- Shoulder issues, 43% of participants could perform athletics for less than 10 minutes prior to prolotherapy. Only 12% could after. Another 20% were able to exercise without restriction.
- Knee issues, 50% of participants could perform athletics for less than 10 minutes prior to prolotherapy. Only 12% could after. Another 38% were able to exercise without restriction.
- Low back, 45% of participants could perform athletics for less than 10 minutes prior to prolotherapy. Only 12% could after. Another 21% were able to exercise without restriction.
- Hip issues, 37% of participants could perform athletics for less than 10 minutes prior to prolotherapy. Only 11% could after. Another 24% were able to exercise without restriction.

I am depressed. Will this help me get my life back?
51-59% of participants were not depressed prior to receiving prolotherapy, this improved to between 84-90% of participants not being depressed after prolotherapy. 25-39% regained a life free from depression.

Is RIT safe?

In the Journal Of Orthopaedic Medicine 1993;15:28-32

T. Dorman wrote: Prolotherapy A Survey. 494,845 patients surveyed, 343,897 for low back, only 66 minor complications: 24 allergic reactions, 29 pneumothorax, and 14 major complications: defined as a patient hospitalization or transient or permanent nerve damage.

This is a complication rate of .016%.

In order to optimize your response to prolotherapy you need a good strong immune system (so their body can lay down the collagen necessary to heal), a willingness to comply with recommended treatment protocol, a positive mental outlook and a healthy diet that will promote healing.

Prolotherapy will not get an optimal result when the patient has a depressed immune system (their body cannot respond to the proliferants), nutritional deficiencies or even nutrient allergies, hormonal deficiencies or excess (increased cortisol from stress can negate healing). The body may be slow to heal especially in our older patients who may need IV vitamins, minerals and other nutrients to augment therapy. At times the wrong area is treated (could be ankle causing knee pain, low back pain caused by knee pain, etc.). The cause of hip and low back pain can be hard to differentiate. It possibly be from the hip, low back or both.

For the person who has many other health challenges, these typically need to be addressed first for RIT to be successful. **Note: patients who are taking Blood thinners cannot be treated.**

Will insurance cover these treatments?

This depends entirely on the coverage your insurance provides.

For more information please refer to the Journal of Prolotherapy http://www.journalofprolotherapy.com

References

1. Journal Of Orthopaedic Medicine 1993;15:28-32

2. Ross A. Hauser, MD; Marion A. Hauser, MS, RD; Joseph J. Cukla, BA, LPN. A Retrospective Observational Study on Hackett-Hemwall Dextrose Prolotherapy for Unresolved Foot and Toe Pain at an Outpatient Charity Clinic in Rural Illinois Journal Of Prolotherapy. volume 3 , issue 1, February 2011

3. Ross A. Hauser, MD; Nicole M. Baird, CHFP; Joe J. Cukla, LPN. A Retrospective Observational Study on Hackett-Hemwall Dextrose Prolotherapy for Unresolved Hand and Finger Pain. Journal Of Prolotherapy Volume 2 , Issue 4 P480 November 2010

4. Ross A. Hauser, MD & Marion A. Hauser, MS, RD. A Retrospective Study on Hackett-Hemwall Dextrose Prolotherapy for Chronic Shoulder Pain. Journal Of Prolotherapy Volume 1 , Issue 4 P214 November 2009

5. Ross A. Hauser, MD & Marion A. Hauser, MS, RD. A Retrospective Study on Dextrose Prolotherapy for Unresolved Knee Pain. Journal Of Prolotherapy Volume 1 , Issue 1 February 2009

6. Ross A. Hauser, MD & Marion A. Hauser, MS, RD. Dextrose Prolotherapy for Unresolved Low Back Pain. Journal Of Prolotherapy Volume 1 , Issue 3 P145 August 2009

7. Ross A. Hauser, MD & Marion A. Hauser, MS, RD. A Retrospective Study on Hackett-Hemwall Dextrose Prolotherapy for Chronic Hip Pain. Journal Of Prolotherapy Volume 1 , Issue 2, P76-88 May 2009

Supplements

Nutrients are necessary for every structure and function in the body. A nutrient is defined as a chemical substance that provides energy, forms new components or assists in various bodily processes. In today's busy world it is difficult to find healthy foods, ensure a clean environment or live completely stress free. Health supplements are an intervention that can easily be integrated into our busy lives.

Nutrition was only recognized as a distinct discipline in 1934, almost 200 years after the first nutritional experiment. A British physician, Dr. James Lind, studied the effect of foods containing ascorbic acid (Vitamin C) on scurvy. The Royal Navy adopted his recommendations several decades after his discovery. Eventually, the Royal Navy decreed that a certain amount of citrus fruit must be kept on board for each sailor. The absence of scurvy was a contributing factor to the British rule of the high seas and their nickname 'limey'.

Despite his success in 1747, the concept of vitamins as necessary bodily nutrients was only discovered in 1912 by Casimir Funk. He proposed that pellagra, beriberi, scurvy and rickets were diseases of deficiency and not caused by a bacteria. Funk knew that "vital for life" nutrients with a nitrogen component could correct the deficiency, thus leading to the term "vita-mine" (*vita* meaning "essential for life" in Latin and *amine* for "nitrogen containing compound"). Eventually the "e" was removed following the realization that not all vitamins contained nitrogen, creating the word we use today "vitamin".

Modern health supplements supply critical nutrients to compensate for common deficiencies, genetics, toxic build-up, enzyme defects and to prevent or treat illnesses. Supplements have the potential to play a major role in health and can be easily used as a complementary treatment in many cases.

Dietary deficiency:
Micronutrients are being consumed in minimal amounts today compared to our ancestors. The average diet is significantly lacking essential nutrients. The nutrient content of food has shifted due to the focus of modern farming techniques on producing higher yields. From 1940-2000, nutrient content has declined significantly: magnesium 21-35%, potassium 6-14%, calcium 16-29%, iron 15-32%, copper 81%, riboflavin (B2) 38% and vitamin C 15%.

Absorption defects:
Not only does our food contain fewer nutrients, but gastrointestinal disturbances can contribute to malabsorption and hereditary absorption defects. Folic acid, biotin, magnesium and zinc are some of the common poorly absorbed nutrients. Absorption is essential to supplementation. Taking a handful of pills daily is not effective if your body is not able to metabolize them properly. At

NaturoMedic.com we seek to correct this prior to supplementation to ensure that you will absorb your nutrients properly.

Enzyme defects:
Supplementation has been demonstrated to improve body function for at least 50 inherited enzyme defects. This includes conversion of a vitamin to its active form.

Disease deficiencies:
The body's nutrient requirements can be altered by the presence of disease especially if the illness causes an increased metabolic rate, such as hyperthyroidism (depleting vitamins A, B, C, E, copper, iron). In the case of congestive heart failure, the heart tissue faces an impaired ability to absorb magnesium, potassium, calcium, zinc, vitamin C and B vitamins.

Drug-induced deficiencies:
Certain medications are capable of promoting nutrient deficiencies. Supplementation can be beneficial in preventing drug side effects.

Nutritional requirements for the general population are often calculated by taking the mean (average) requirement hence the Recommended Dietary Allowances (RDA). Other factors including safety, exposure, stress and nutrient stability are taken into consideration too. Unfortunately, there are downfalls to the RDAs. These values are established for a healthy population and do not take into account disease states (digestive difficulties, malabsorption, chronic infection), genetic defects, environmental pollutants or increased need due to medications. These are special instances that would increase a person's RDA. Considering how wide spread disease trends have become, we recognize that the RDAs should be considered as general guidelines. Each person has an individual optimal requirement that will likely fall well above the RDA and well below the toxic dose. Your NaturoMedic.com Naturopathic Doctor will recommend the most appropriate and safest dose for your nutritional supplementation, taking into account the most recent research and the effectiveness of various nutrients.

References:
1.   Marz, R. Medical Nutrition. 2nd edition. 2002. Omni-Press. Portland, OR.
2.   Gaby, A. Nutritional Medicine. 2011. Fritz Perlberg Publishing. Concord, NH.
3.   Pizzorno, J & Murray, M. Textbook of Natural Medicine. 3rd edition. 2006. Elsevier Ltd. Churchill Livingstone. St. Louis, Missouri.
4.   http://www.agelessway.org/whyusehenusu.html

Trigger Point Injections & Neural Therapy

Trigger Point Injection Therapy

Trigger Point Injection (TPI) therapy is a procedure designed to relieve pain in areas of muscle that contain knots. Knots, classified as trigger points are discrete, hyperirritable spots (feel like a rope) located in a tight band of muscle. These points can often be felt under the skin and they produce pain locally. This irritates the nerves around them and in a referred pattern to other areas of the body. Acute trauma or repetitive stress on muscle fibers can lead to the formation of trigger points. Persistent pain can occur in postural muscles in the neck, shoulders and pelvis. Palpation over a trigger point will also elicit pain directly over the area or the radiation of pain in the body. Many disorders can result following trigger point formation including tension headaches, tinnitus, jaw pain, low back pain, arm pain, shoulder pain, leg pain and decreased range of motion.

Trigger Point Injection is used to treat many muscle groups throughout the body. It has been used successfully to treat fibromyalgia and myofascial pain syndrome (chronic pain involving tissue that surrounds the muscle). A needle is inserted directly into the trigger point injecting pain alleviating solutions such as lidocaine or procaine. These restore function to the autonomic nervous system and allow the muscle to relax. By relaxing the spasming muscle, blood flow to the area is improved and the trigger point is inactivated. Solutions including homeopathics and B vitamins may also be used for injection. TPI has a variety of benefits including immediate and long-lasting relief of pain, reduced referred pain and minimized fatigue and stiffness. Several sites may be injected in one visit providing sustained relief.

Neural Therapy

Neural therapy was originally developed in Germany to provide instant and long-lasting resolution of chronic pain and illness. The therapy is based on the theory that trauma can produce disturbances in the electrochemical function of tissues. Areas of trauma, for example scar tissue, have different membrane charges then normal body cells. In other words, your cells are similar to a battery. If the charge on the battery changes, abnormal minerals and toxic substances can accumulate as the pumps in the wall of the cell stop working. Consequently, the cell can no longer heal itself. In neural therapy, a local anesthetic, such as procaine, is injected to restore the functioning of the pumps and normal membrane potential (correct the charge on the battery). By re-establishing the appropriate electrical condition of the cell, the disturbed function is neutralized allowing you to return to health. Solutions including homeopathics and B vitamins may also be used for injection.

Similar to TPI, the site being treated can affect other areas in the body. A scar on the arm can affect your back due to the vast nerve network in our body. We are basically connected by one large electrical circuit. TPI is a type of neural therapy; however neural therapy can be used for additional conditions such as allergies, bowel dysfunction, menstrual irregularities, infertility, etc. Neural therapy can have a profound impact on your condition and your ability to heal.

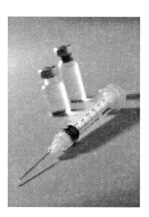

References:

1. http://www.aafp.org/afp/2002/0215/p653.html
2. http://www.medicinenet.com/trigger_point_injection/article.htm
3. http://www.fibromyalgia-symptoms.org/fibromyalgia_injections.html
4. http://www.drkaslow.com/html/neural_therapy.html

The Q2 Water Energy System

Q2 therapy is based on the principle that all living things produce a form of organic electricity or Bio-Charge. The Q2 system produces a complex electromagnetic waveform that resonates throughout the water and interacts synergistically with the bioelectric state of the body. Absorption of this bio-charge has been shown to increase the potential voltage of the body's cell membranes, helping to maintain cellular function. The magnetic technology of the Q2 permeates and realigns your energy field.

Benefits of the Q2:

- Increased vitality, energy and overall well-being
- Enhanced recovery time
- Revitalized blood
- Detoxification and neutralization of toxins
- Improved sleeping patterns
- Pain and stress relief
- Reduced inflammation
- Dermal (skin) rejuvenation
- Improved internal organ function, including kidney and liver function
- Improved metabolic and endocrine function
- Reduced fluid retention
- Elimination of menstrual pain
- Improved concentration

Water is necessary to convert the electrical charge emitted by the Q2 metal rings into a bio charge. By having your feet immersed in water with a Q2 Unit, the bio-charge produced will amplify your own personal healthy frequencies. The bio-charge boost can help restore your system to optimum function.

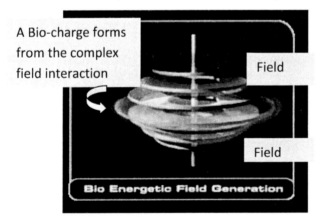

A Bio-charge forms from the complex field interaction

Field

Field

Bio Energetic Field Generation

During the immersion process, the Q2 stimulates the release of foreign materials and toxins from the body. This often can result in added discoloration of water, however please note that most of the colour change is due to the presence of minerals that precipitate out during electrolysis from the Q2 metal rings. In other words, the electric charge from the plates separates minerals already present in the water and which initiates the colour change.

Method of Use

With both of your feet immersed in a large basin of water, the Q2 orb is placed into the water. The Q2 unit is turned on for approximately 35 minutes. All you need to do is sit back and relax. You may read or have a light snack during your treatments. The frequencies of your treatments will depend on what the doctor has suggested for your individual care. However, it is recommended that treatments be completed every other day for a period of one month.

Who should not use the Q2 Energy Spa?

The Q2 is not recommended for use by anyone with battery operated implants such as pacemakers. If you are pregnant or if you have any organs implanted it is also not recommended.

References:
1. http://www.braintuner.com/befe.htm
2. http://healthandlight.com/q2_benefits.htm

VT-15: Vibration Therapy

Whole body vibration (WBV) is a beneficial technology that has been released to the public in recent years. This therapy can gently and safely improve your health, well-being and overall fitness. The benefit of vibration was first mentioned as treatment in ancient Greece for the Olympians. They realized they could enhance muscle performance by wrapping a saw in cotton and then running the saw back and forth over the body in the target area. Today's technology has advanced beyond the use of a saw and closely resembles the vibration exercise that was created in 1960 by a Russian Scientist in Germany. The therapy was used to rehabilitate Cosmonauts after returning from space to repair atrophied muscles and bone density loss. The most discussed example was in 1995 when Valery Polakov, a Russian Cosmonaut, set a World Record for being in space for 438 days. Due to vibration technology, American astronauts typically only went for 120 days. This therapy was quickly embraced by NASA shortly after and led to the development of Whole Body Vibration platforms.

The VT-15 Vibration Platform produces vertical vibrations from a side alternating rocking movement which simulates walking as you stand. The energy is transferred to your body and stimulates every cell, muscle, bone and soft tissue. The body reacts to this movement with an involuntary reflex and, depending on the set speed of the machine; your muscles will contract up to 23 times per second (approx. 11-12 contractions and relaxations per second). The body will feel as if it weighs more as acceleration increases. You work against a greater load of gravity in every movement, but it puts less stress on joints, ligaments and tendons compared to regular resistance training. As a result, you achieve more benefits in less time. During your session the entire body is stimulated by the vibrations, working every area at once instead of one muscle group at a time with a standard weight workout. A 10-minute workout may be similar to 1 hour at the gym. There are also vertical vibration machines available. For instance, Dr. Mercola recommends a tri-directional machine that oscillates side to side, forward and back, as well as vertically. This vertical movement is very intense and places a great deal of load on the body potentially leading to long term compression injuries and limiting its use to people who are already quite physically fit. Be aware of which type of machine you are using.

There are a variety of health benefits to vibration therapy. They can include:

- muscle toning and strengthening in 3 weeks
- increased bone density in 6-8 weeks
- increased production of serotonin
- endorphins and testosterone

- decreased cortisol and cellulite
- tightening of skin
- lower blood pressure
- increased metabolism and fat-burning
- increased blood circulation
- increased flexibility
- mobility and co-ordination
- improved balance
- increased lymphatic drainage
- assists in detoxification
- relief of stress, headaches, joint and back pain

WBV has been used to treat osteoporosis and osteoarthritis, incontinence, peripheral neuropathy, depression and Parkinson's. It has also been recommended to improve recovery from injury after surgery. The speed of the vibrations directly influences the desired benefit. In general low speeds are ideal for posture and strength, middle speeds for weight training and stretching and finally higher speeds for massage and muscle relaxation.

References:
1. http://www.tzonevibrationtech.com/technology.html
2. http://www.mayoclinic.com/health/whole-body-vibration/AN01598
3. http://www.wholebodyvibrationsystem.com/Theamazingwellnessbenefits.pdf

Summary

The Health Navigator is designed to expose the many potholes and obstacles impeding your journey to your health destination. Goal setting and an effective health strategy are mandatory for success in your endeavor. As the Navigator tools teach you how to conquer the challenges of health on your road through life, they also establish the benefit of accountability and commitment. At NaturoMedic.com, our integrated health strategy incorporates 5 key principles to expedite results and uphold persistence.

Thank you for taking the initial steps to learn about your health and work towards being blessed with good health.

We have empowered you with the knowledge you need to navigate the way through your journey of well-being. This strategy will remove the burdens of the Environment, Lifestyle, Body, Mind and Spirit to progress through The Health Continuum™ to health optimization. What you do with this wealth of knowledge is up to you; the ball is now in your court! With this in mind, we return to our original questions: **what are your health goals and do you have a health strategy?**

Spread the word and be a leader of health. Your voyage will continue throughout life, but the story of your success will always be invaluable.

The NaturoMedic.com Team

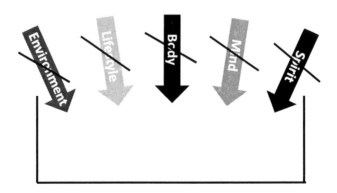